EYE AND VISION RESEARCH DEVELOPMENTS

NOVEL DRUG DELIVERY APPROACHES IN DRY EYE SYNDROME THERAPY

EYE AND VISION RESEARCH DEVELOPMENTS

Additional books in this series can be found on Nova's website under the Series tab.

Additional E-books in this series can be found on Nova's website under the E-book tab.

EYE AND VISION RESEARCH DEVELOPMENTS

NOVEL DRUG DELIVERY APPROACHES IN DRY EYE SYNDROME THERAPY

ELIANA B. SOUTO
SLAVOMIRA DOKTOROVOVÁ
JOANA R. ARAÚJO
MARIA A. EGEA
AND
MARIA L. GARCIA

Nova Biomedical
Nova Science Publishers, Inc.
New York

Copyright © 2010 by Nova Science Publishers, Inc.

All rights reserved. No part of this book may be reproduced, stored in a retrieval system or transmitted in any form or by any means: electronic, electrostatic, magnetic, tape, mechanical photocopying, recording or otherwise without the written permission of the Publisher.

For permission to use material from this book please contact us:
Telephone 631-231-7269; Fax 631-231-8175
Web Site: http://www.novapublishers.com

NOTICE TO THE READER

The Publisher has taken reasonable care in the preparation of this book, but makes no expressed or implied warranty of any kind and assumes no responsibility for any errors or omissions. No liability is assumed for incidental or consequential damages in connection with or arising out of information contained in this book. The Publisher shall not be liable for any special, consequential, or exemplary damages resulting, in whole or in part, from the readers' use of, or reliance upon, this material.

Independent verification should be sought for any data, advice or recommendations contained in this book. In addition, no responsibility is assumed by the publisher for any injury and/or damage to persons or property arising from any methods, products, instructions, ideas or otherwise contained in this publication.

This publication is designed to provide accurate and authoritative information with regard to the subject matter covered herein. It is sold with the clear understanding that the Publisher is not engaged in rendering legal or any other professional services. If legal or any other expert assistance is required, the services of a competent person should be sought. FROM A DECLARATION OF PARTICIPANTS JOINTLY ADOPTED BY A COMMITTEE OF THE AMERICAN BAR ASSOCIATION AND A COMMITTEE OF PUBLISHERS.

Library of Congress Cataloging-in-Publication Data

Novel drug delivery approaches in dry eye syndrome therapy / authors, Slavomira Doktorovova ... [et al.].
   p. ; cm.
Includes bibliographical references and index.
ISBN 978-1-61668-768-7 (softcover)
1. Dry eye syndromes--Chemotherapy. 2. Ophthalmic drugs. 3. Drugs--Dosage forms. I. Doktorovova, Slavomira.
[DNLM: 1. Dry Eye Syndromes--drug therapy. 2. Drug Delivery Systems. 3. Lacrimal Apparatus Diseases--drug therapy. WW 208 N937 2010]
RE216.D78N68 2010
617.7'15--dc22
                        2010015613

Published by Nova Science Publishers, Inc. ✦ New York

Contents

Preface		vii
Authors' Contact Information		ix
Abbreviations		11
Chapter I	Introduction	13
Chapter II	Lachrymal Functional Unit and Dry Eye Syndrome	17
Chapter III	Therapeutic Approaches of the Dry Eye Syndrome	23
Chapter IV	Conclusions and Future Trends	43
References		47
Index		61

Preface

Dry eye syndrome or the *keratoconjunctivitis sicca* is a common disease of tear film and ocular surface developed in numerous aetiologies. Tear film instability and ocular surface disturbances that subsequently influence the tear film are among the primarily causes of this disease, but many other factors are involved in tear film disorders. Clinical manifestations commonly include eye discomfort, feeling of a foreign body in the eye, itching or even visual disturbance; inflammation and damage of ocular surface may follow. The therapeutic approaches are based on the dry eye symptoms relief, increasing the patient's comfort and preventing further damage to ocular surface. This can be achieved by renewing the normal function of tear film and ocular surfaces. Although eye surface is easily reached by classical ocular dosage forms, novel drug delivery systems for ocular administration offer advantages in terms of increased residence time on eye surface and/or controlled release of the drug, with enhanced therapeutic effectiveness. Patient's acceptance can also be improved by developing formulations that do not require frequent application, or cause blurred vision, and having a more pleasant appearance. Biodegradable, biocompatible, non-toxic, and mucoadhesive materials are being used for the design of colloidal carriers. Novel polymers for hydrogels suitable for ocular administration are reviewed in this chapter, giving overview on their potential benefits and limitations in dry eye syndrome management and reported successful formulations.

Authors' Contact Information

Eliana B. Souto[1,2]
[1] Faculty of Health Sciences, Fernando Pessoa University,
Rua Carlos da Maia, Nr. 296, Office S.1, P-4200-150
Porto, Portugal
Phone: +351-225-074630; Fax: +351-225-074637
Corresponding author: Email: eliana@ufp.edu.pt

[2] Centre of Genetics and Biotechnology,
University of Trás-os-Montes and
Alto Douro (IBB/CGB-UTAD), P.O. Box 1013, 5000-801
Vila Real, Portugal

Slavomira Doktorovová
Centre of Genetics and Biotechnology,
University of Trás-os-Montes and
Alto Douro (IBB/CGB-UTAD), P.O. Box 1013, 5000-801
Vila Real, Portugal

Joana R. Araújo, Maria A. Egea, Maria L. Garcia
Department of Physical Chemistry,
Institute of Nanoscience and
Nanotechnology, Faculty of Pharmacy,
University of Barcelona, Av. Joan XXIII s/n, 08028
Barcelona, Spain

Abbreviations

AUC	Area Under the Curve
KCS	Keratoconjunctivitis Sicca
NC	Nanocapsules
NE	Nanoemulsion
NLC	Nanostructured Lipid Carriers
NP	Nanoparticles
NS	Nanospheres
NSAIDs	Non Steroidal Anti-Inflammatory Drugs
PECL	Poly-ε-caprolactone
PEG	Polyethylene glycol
PIBCA	Poly-isobutyl-cyanoacrylate
PLGA	Poly(lactic-co-glycolic)acid
PVA	Polyvinyl alcohol
RCE	Rabbit Corneal Epithelium
SLN	Solid Lipid Nanoparticles

Chapter I

Introduction

For many decades, *keratoconjunctivitis sicca* (KCS) or dry eye ocular surface disease, was thought to be limited to dryness of the eyes caused by a reduction of the aqueous phase of the tear film. Now it is understood that this definition does not adequately describe the full clinical picture of dry eye disease, while it is true that the most frequent cause of common dry eye is lachrymal hyposecretion, deviations in tear composition also play a decisive role. As such, the modern definition of dry eye disease is based on the concept of the three layers of the tear film devised by Holly and Lemp [1], which can be directly affected by different stimuli, causing qualitative and quantitative changes. The term "dry eye" is generically used to describe a variety of ocular disorders of diverse pathogenesis that share signs of ocular surface abnormalities and symptoms of discomfort, feeling of dryness, grittiness, and/or foreign body sensation.

Most people experience acute dry eye episodes multiple times during lifetime. Prolonged exposure to dry air (e.g., on a long-haul flight), or to a strong current of air from driving at high speed readily induces transient dry eye even in people with healthy eyes. While these common conditions are harmless and are easily resolve spontaneously, chronic dry eye syndrome can severely impair the patients' quality of life and vocational performance. In severe cases that are left untreated, damage to the cornea may result.

Dry eye syndrome is a superficial eye disorder, meaning that the target site of the drug is the external tissues of the eye. The optimal ocular dosage form suitable for use in dry eye syndrome management should enable the delivery of the actives to the relevant ocular tissue ideally without compromising the irrelevant sites. No systemic uptake of the administered drug should occur. As dry eye syndrome is such a common disease, the use of the final product should at the same time be as convenient as possible for the patient, i.e. should be handled easily, and should not interfere with normal vision, therefore not causing any unpleasant sensation upon administration.

The corneal surface can be easily reached by classical ocular dosage forms like eye drops, aqueous suspensions of drugs, hydrogels, or ophthalmic ointments. Eye drops are the most common ocular dosage forms, ideal for instillation of hydrophilic drugs, offering several advantages including easy manipulation, easy manufacture, and low production costs. The well known limitation is the fast elimination of the aqueous dispersion form the ocular surface by blinking and by tear drainage, not allowing the drug to stay onto the ocular surface for sufficient time. Only a low percentage of the drug will permeate the cornea and reach its site of action within the eye.

Ophthalmic hydrogel formulations are an alternative to eye drops that might provide increased residence time of the drug onto the ocular surface. Despite the transparency, blurring of the vision still may occur. Despite blurred vision is not a serious side effect, the patient's comfort and subsequent compliance may be compromised. Another issue of hydrogel formulations is their higher production costs in comparison to eye drops or ocular ointments.

Many of the actives relevant in dry eye syndrome management are poorly water soluble. The marketed formulations for this kind of drugs include aqueous suspensions of the drug (e.g., Pred Forte™ with 1% prednisolone acetate from Allergan; Alrex™ with 0.2% loteprednol etabonate from Bausch & Lomb) or ophthalmic emulsions (e.g., Restasis™ with 0.05% cyclosporine from Allergan; Durezol™ with 0.05% difluprednate from Sirion Therapeutics). Achieving therapeutic concentrations of the drugs by means of these forms may also be difficult.

Besides practical advantages and well established usage of these classical ocular dosage forms, there is still a space for improvements in terms of bioavailability, targeted delivery of actives to the desired tissues and controlled release. The aims of employing novel dosage forms include: (i) elimination of possible side effects of the drugs or adverse reactions to the formulations constituents; (ii) improvement of drug bioavailability at the required site of action; (iii) provide prolonged therapeutic effect; (iv) assure convenient application of the medicinal product, preferentially in the form of eye drops; (v) to avoid interfering with vision, i.e. be transparent and show a refractive index similar to that of the tears.

As the cornea contains many nerve endings, the size of the carriers that might be used in ophthalmic formulations without causing the sensation of foreign body in the eye and itching is limited to particle diameters below 1 μm [2]. Some authors prefer even smaller particle size for ocular drug delivery e.g. below 500 nm [3] Therefore, any drug carrier intended for ocular administration should have diameter within this size range. Nanoparticle formulations prepared from various materials are being proposed as alternative drug formulation by many research teams. Apart from the suitable size, further reasons for using nanoparticle-based formulation in ocular drug delivery are: (i) the possibility to be applied onto the ocular surface in the same way as eye drops (as aqueous nanoparticle dispersions); (ii) their submicron meter size of the particles avoiding interfering with the vision; and (iii) the possibility to provide a controlled release of the active. Prolonged release of actives is often achieved by encapsulation of the actives into various carriers. The drug must however release from the carrier in such a time that allows its further penetration into the target tissue before the carrier is eliminated from the site.

Chapter II

Lachrymal Functional Unit and Dry Eye Syndrome

Tear secretion is controlled and coordinated by the lachrymal functional unit, composed of the main and accessory lachrymal glands, the ocular surface (cornea, conjunctiva and meibomian glands) and the interconnecting innervations. Subconscious stimulation of the free nerve endings populating the cornea, results in the generation of afferent nerve impulses through the ophthalmic branch of the trigeminal nerve on to the mid-brain where they synapse, signal is integrated and sent by efferent branch of the loop through the pterygopalatine ganglion to the lachrymal glands [4].

The eyelids, which serve as a protective device for the eye, moisten the surface of the cornea by producing a tear film of 10 μm thick that prevents desiccation. This tear film consists of three layers: (i) a superficial lipid layer mainly composed of wax and cholesteryl esters and some polar lipids, which plays a major role in maintaining that function; (ii) the aqueous layer, which is important to the maintain the corneal transparency; and a mucous layer sticking to the epithelial cells, responsible for the adherence of the tear film to the cornea. Another essential task of the conjunctiva is the immunological defence provided by Langerhans cells and lymphatic follicles which contain T and B lymphocytes, various subtypes of reticular cells and macrophages.

Tears are also important in wound healing, by providing a pathway by which blood cells make their way from the circulation into central corneal openings, and in the aerobic metabolism of the corneal epithelium, obtaining and dissolving oxygen from the atmosphere. The normal tear quantity, its anti-inflammatory constituents and the secretion of mucin, repair and prevent damage during exposure of the ocular surface in a normal individual to environmental stresses such as wind, low humidity, blinking, or exposure of the surface to bacteria, viruses or particles.

2.1. Causes of the Dry Eye

A number of ocular surface conditions may trigger dry eye disease or be associated with it. Evidence indicates that chronic dry eye results from a T cell-mediated inflammatory pathology [5]. The ocular surface, lachrymal glands, and interconnecting nerves form a homeostatic functional unit that maintains normal tear production and multiple factors, including an age-related drop in systemic androgen levels, autoimmune disorders such as Sjögren's syndrome, or meibomian gland dysfunction, create an environment in which activated T cells are recruited to the ocular surface and lachrymal glands, disrupting the normal nerve traffic and perpetuating a cycle of immune-based inflammation that ultimately results in destruction of the lachrymal glands [6]. Environmental factors such as hot climates, pollution, the use of visual display terminals and contact lenses may also cause chronic ocular surface irritation that can contribute to the onset of dry eye symptoms [7].

Pharmacological and toxic dry eye has been known since the last century. Drugs reported as being relevant for the reduction of lachrymal secretion are atropine, contraceptives, antiestrogen tamoxifen, tranquilizers, acetylsalicylic acid, the antineoplasic busulfan, the antiangina pectoris perhexiline, alpha-adrenergic stimulants and beta-adrenergic blockers. Some toxic chemicals may also desiccate the eye (denaturalized colza oil, botulinum toxin, typhoid fever) [8]. Vitamin A is essential for maintaining the health of epithelial cells throughout the body, affecting cellular regulation and differentiation [9], its deficiency adversely affects epithelial cells. Thus, an absence of this active causes the loss of goblet cells and leads to increased epidermal keratinization and squamous metaplasia of the mucous membranes, generally including the cornea and conjunctiva [10]. This type of avitaminose due to malnutrition in underdeveloped countries and other nutritional conditions such as hyponutrition, alcoholism and dehydration, is also accepted as causes of dry eye.

Sjögren's syndrome, named after the Swedish ophthalmologist Henrik Sjögren, was first described it in 1933, as a chronic autoimmune rheumatic disorder characterized by lymphocytic infiltration of exocrine glands and mucosae [11], leading to destruction of the glandular tissue. Lymphocyte diapedesis and homing to ocular tissues are induced and regulated by multiple signalling pathways. During the initial phase of cell response to injury, immune or inflammatory insults, the corneal and conjunctival epithelial cells can be stimulated to express inflammatory molecules such as cytokines and cell adhesion molecules [12, 13]. Chemokines, a family of chemotactic cytokines that signal through G-protein coupled receptors, and Inter Cellular Adhesion Molecule-1 (ICAM-1), one of the most important intercellular adhesion molecules, will in turn promote lymphocyte activation and further recruitment to the ocular tissues and lachrymal glands [14]. As a result, inflammation will occur within the lachrymal functional unit leading towards an alteration in tear quantity and composition, interrupting neuronal reflex signalling and exacerbating inflammation manifestation. The loss of neural function results in sensory isolation of the lachrymal glands and the elimination of requisite neural tone, as a consequence lachrymal glands atrophy, presenting cellular breakdown proteins to the cell surface. Apoptosis (i.e., programmed cell death) of T lymphocytes is a gene-regulated process that functions abnormally in patients with Sjögren's syndrome and appears to contribute to glandular destruction and an altered tear film [15].

Besides the association with Sjögren's syndrome exocrinopathy, dry eye may also be associated with several endocrinopathies, Graves-Basedow's disease, diabetes mellitus, pheochromocytoma, ovariectomy, premature ovarian failure, hypothyroidism and various conditions involving the menstrual cycle, menopause, pregnancy and involution senilis [8].

In patients with atopic dermatitis, which is another skin and mucosae disorder or autoimmune connective tissue disease, KCS is a severe and often chronic ocular surface inflammatory condition, occurring conjunctival scarring and corneal complications, leading to significant visual morbidity. Viral infections, such as infectious mononucleosis, cytomegalovirus, AIDS and viral keratoconjunctivitis (e.g., *Bacillus xerosis*) have also been considered causes of dry eye due to an immune response or to direct involvement of the lachrymal glands. Immunopathological changes include invasion of the epithelium by eosinophils and mast cells and significant infiltration of the stroma by activated T-cells that produce IL-2 and IFN-γ [16, 17].

Changes in the hormonal environment surrounding the ocular surface and lachrymal gland is one of the key factors involved in the etiology of KCS. The common hormonal status in female populations of non-Sjögren's KCS is a decrease in circulating androgens due to decreased function of the ovaries in the post-menopausal woman, and also to secretion of sex hormone binding globulin during pregnancy and birth control pill use [18, 19]. Therefore, it is believed that androgens provide trophic support of the lachrymal gland as well as meibomian gland function and its deficiency or inherent insensitivity may lead to meibomian gland disease [20, 21]

Apoptosis is a series of physiological events in the cell which ensure the balance between cell division and loss, therefore contributing for the regulation of tissue development and homeostasis. Pathological apoptosis may also happen, if abnormal increase and/or decrease in the rate of apoptotic cell death in target tissues occurs. Such condition has been demonstrated in various types of diseases including dry eye. Clinically, apoptosis-related markers were found to be upregulated in conjunctival cells from patients with moderate to severe KCS, with or without Sjögren's syndrome [11], indicating an important role in the pathogenesis of KCS.

Other reason for dry eye symptoms includes neurosensorial deprivation of the lachrymal basin caused by an interruption of the trigeminal nerve. Subsidiary corneal damage due to dryness, scarce or incomplete blinking, traumatic aggression or a lack of neurotrophic stimuli results in the release of pro-inflammatory neural transmitters such as substance P. This neuropeptide enhance the activation status of vigilant lymphocytes and the release of cytokines leading to neurogenic inflammation symptoms [22].

Despite the plurality of the underlying causes of dry eye, there are several common histopathologic manifestations of the ocular surface epithelia, namely, the loss of the conjunctival goblet cells, abnormal enlargement of the epithelial cells, increase in cellular stratification, and keratinization [23]. The normal secretory conjunctival mucosa gradually develops into a nonsecretory keratinized epithelium, a process referred to as squamous metaplasia [24].

Obstruction of meibomian gland ducts, whether by epithelial squamous metaplasia, chalazia, or solidified lipids, results in decreased secretion of abnormal tear lipids [25]. Lipases originating from bacteria colonizing the lid margin are believed to degrade some of the lipids as they are secreted, changing lipid composition of the tear film. The partially degraded lipids depict high melting point and, therefore, are more likely to solidify and block meibomian gland orifices at body temperature. Changes in lipid layer of the tear film allows increased evaporation of the aqueous component, leading to many of the signs and symptoms found in chronic dry eye [26].

2.2. Signs and Symptoms of the Dry Eye

The most frequent symptoms of dry eye include irritation, sensation of strange body, existence of filamentous mucosity and transitory blurred vision. Other less frequent symptoms are photophobia, sensation of fatigue and slowness of eyelids. All these symptoms can be exacerbated in those situations where an increase of the evaporation takes place (heat, conditioned air or wind) and can improve closing the eyes. In slight to moderate dry eye, patients can have crisis of intense lachrymation, that does not contradict the existence of dry eye, since these crisis can be due to lachrymation reflects (conjuntival or corneal irritation) or emotional reasons, which usually is normal [8].

Often it is possible to suspect of dry eye, only with observing the signs in pre-corneal tearful film, the marginal tearful layer and the own cornea. For pre-corneal film, the increase of mucous fibers can be detected along with the fact that mucin contaminated with lipids is accumulated in the film and moves with the blinking. In the case of the marginal film, this has a reduced height in dry eye (1 mm for healthy eyes), is concave and contains mucosity, in serious cases it can even lack. Others include punctiform epithelial erosions that can be depicted by the cornea; filaments in the form of comma whose free ends hang on the cornea and move with the blinking; mucous plates that pronounce injuries of varied size and formed by epithelial cells, proteins and lipidic substances. Rare but also possible is the corneal perforation in severe cases.

The evaluation of the breakage time of the pre-corneal tearful film is a simple test to diagnose dry eye and is based on the instillation of fluorescein in the inferior sac. The patient is asked to blink several times and stop, one inspects the film with cobalt blue light. After an interval of time, black spots or lines appear in the tear film which indicates the appearance of dry areas. The time of rupture is measured from the last blinking to the appearance of the first dry spot and is considered abnormal when inferior to 10 seconds. Other possible test is the method of Mengher, which uses corneal reflection, clear when the corneal surface is humidified and distortable by dry spots. Projecting on the cornea a square, the clinician can control the time that takes in distorting the square by the first dry spot.

Chapter III

Therapeutic Approaches of the Dry Eye Syndrome

Treatment of the dry eye involves the challenges and frustrations associated with the management of a chronic disease. There is generally no cure but, with proper attention and an adequate treatment regimen, it is likely that good vision can be preserved throughout life and a considerable degree of comfort afforded.

General measures to decrease dryness include reviewing the patient's medications to consider replacing one or more drying agents with medications that have fewer anticholinergic effects. Avoiding environmental factors (e.g., wind, dust, smoke, and low humidity), increasing fluid intake (especially water), avoiding use of excessive eye makeup (particularly on the eyelid, because it can soften and enter the eye, creating more concentrated tears), and using moisture-chamber glasses specifically designed to protect the eye from irritants and hold sponges that increase the humidity surrounding the eye, are measures that may help improving eye comfort.

The main objectives of diverse therapeutic options are to alleviate the pain, contribute to a uniform optical surface, prevent corneal injuries and prevent probable causes of dry eye. Traditional therapies, such as punctal occlusion and artificial tears, are palliative measures that attempt to increase the volume of the tear film by either reducing drainage or supplementing the tear film with an aqueous solution [27]. Important factors in the success of dry eye therapy are the full information of patients about the nature of their disease, the goals of the clinician´s choice and the encouragement of compliance with the regimen.

3.1. Current Therapeutic Strategies

Although the definitive cure remains elusive, a number of measures are available for managing various dry eye manifestations. The most appropriate type of treatment modality for each patient must be carefully studied and proceeded, being determined by the severity of the condition. Further research to identify more completely the pathogenetic mechanisms involved in the development of the dry eye is ongoing. It is hoped that the results of such studies will allow the direction of therapy more specifically and even more successfully in the near future.

3.1.1. Tear Substitution: Artificial Tear Substitutes and Lubricants

The eye's primary line of defence is its tear film, a complex isotonic liquid containing a mixture of proteins (including enzymes such as lysozyme, which dissolves gram-negative bacteria) and lipids. Tear replacement by topical artificial tears and lubricants is currently the most widely used therapy for dry eye, with the goal of increasing humidity and improving lubrication at the ocular surface [6].

Tear film substitution by the use of artificial tears has however some limitations. The complex composition of natural tears is difficult to replace and the ability of lachrymal glands to massively increase tear production in response to the introduction of any irritant onto the ocular surface means that eye drops require isotonic, no irritating, and perhaps even astringent formulations. Otherwise, they will be instantly diluted, and even completely flushed out, before they have a chance to diffuse through the cornea - which in itself acts as a barrier for diffusion. Apart from a good tolerance and high surface stability, an ideal tear substitute requires a long retention period, while not being too viscous, as this would have a negative influence on visual acuity, and as far as possible, it should contain no foreign substances, such as irritating preservatives [28].

Lubricants are aqueous solutions of polymers able to meet the requirements of wetting agents, i.e., hydrophilizing the corneal surface and extending adhesion and retention periods in the eye. Available preparations consisting of semi-synthetic cellulose derivates, polyvinyl alcohol, polyvinylpyrrolidone, polyacrylic acid derivates, dextran or hyaluronic acid aqueous solutions reduce the surface tension of the tear fluid, afford improved corneal moistening, thicken and stabilize the pre-corneal tear film, and consequently allow dry eye symptoms relief. However, they all have limited periods of ocular retention. This requirement can be reached by adding to the formulations, ingredients designed to have mucoadhesive properties. Many of these components are formulated as viscous gels [29], which tend to cause irritation, blur vision, make the eyelid sticky and create a sensation of heavy eyelids. Different formulation strategies can simply use less viscous materials [30], biopolymeric systems that allow less viscosity while retaining mucoadhesive properties [31], or the polymer chitosan, which has bioadhesive and lubricating properties [32-34].

Some patients with KCS have particularly viscous, stringy mucus that may be associated with filaments or coarse mucous plaques on the ocular surface, which appear to be major sources of irritation and discomfort [35, 36]. This condition can be ameliorated by daily application of mucolytic solutions, such as 10 to 20% solutions of acetylcysteine 4 to 5 times.

Lipids are usually formulated as ointments which are usually an inconvenience in KCS, since these formulations are not able to mix with the tear film and may damage the pre-corneal film. As a result, these formulations may drastically reduce the breakup time i.e., breaking the tear film within a few seconds when the eye is open. However, there are some preservative-free formulations on the market that can provide relief for patients experiencing symptoms of insufficient moistening action during the night and upon awakening, their application provides a long-lasting means of increasing lubricity between the eyelid and the ocular surface during sleep [35, 36].

To obtain a continuous and adequate treatment, repeated application is required. For this, ophthalmic preparations in multiple-dose containers are necessary and applications from such containers are subject to contamination, being iatrogenic infections with Pseudomonas aeruginosa the most problematic [37]. To ensure a long shelf-life and stability of preparations in multiple-dose containers, in addition to polymers manufacturers commonly employ a variety of stabilizers and preservatives. The most currently used preservatives are quaternary ammonium compounds (benzalkonium chloride, benzododecinium bromide, cetrimide, polyquad), alcohols (chlorobutanol) and other compounds (e.g., chlorhexidine, sorbic acid, potassium sorbate, boric acid, biguanides), acting primarily against the bacterial cell membrane, damaging or destroying it [38-40]. Nevertheless, one must bear in mind that all preservatives have more or less pronounced irritating properties and citotoxicity in the cells of the ocular surface. As such, single-dose preservative-free containers are a suitable alternative to patients having to apply ophthalmic formulations frequently and for extended periods. The drawbacks presented by these single unit-dose tears are the high cost and the induced lack of compliance, because patients must carry numerous vials to maintain adequate dosage over the day.

Other common additives used in artificial tear preparations are buffers, which have the purpose of maintaining the pH of human natural tears as closely as possible when they are applied [38, 39]. As a rule, slightly alkaline isotonic or almost isotonic moistening agents are preferred in KCS treatment, as they seem to be more comfortable than neutral or acidic preparations. Accordingly, most commercially available tear substitutes are maintained at a pH value between 7.23 and 7.5 by bicarbonates, phosphates, acetates, citrates, borates and sodium hydroxide.

Another important factor is tear film osmolarity, which is also an irritative factor [41]. In general, its value ranges between 303 and 305 mosm/L and in patients with dry eye this is increased up to 30-40 mosm/L. consequently the attempt is to reduce this increased osmolarity by applying hypotonic electrolyte-based formulations [42, 43]. Bicarbonate seems to be an essential electrolyte in the recovery of the damaged corneal epithelial barrier and in the maintenance of normal ultrastructure [44].

When conditions of dry eye are mild, a tear substitute with low viscosity is recommended, as far as possible no more often than four times per day. In cases of more pronounced dry eye, the frequency of eye drop application must be increased to ten times per day. Besides, the application of commercially available tear substitutes is frequently insufficient for patients with severe forms of KCS, and a too frequent use may result in toxic or allergic reactions due to the cumulative effect of the preservatives. These patients prefer inserts, since these are small, solid, yet soft polymers introduced into the cul-de-sac which, suffer continuous moistening by the natural tear fluid, take several hours to dissolve, and avoid frequent drop applications. The first sustained-release artificial tear inserts becoming available (Lacriserts™) were 5 mg hydroxypropyl cellulose rods that dissolve on contact with the ocular surface, releasing a viscous watery coating that can last 6 to 12 hours [45]. Although being preservative free and used only twice a day, they have the disadvantages of being expensive, difficult to manage, producing the sensation of a foreign body present in the eye and may occasionally cause mild striated vision while being dissolved. Related to this system is a new preservative-free lyophilised drug delivery system with better tolerability, in which hydroxypropylmethyl cellulose detaches from a polymeric carrier upon contact with the tear film [46].

Surgical procedures aiming to substitute tears by fluids from other exocrine glands offers an alternative to the most difficult cases [47]. The parotid salivary gland is a choice being its outward duct transplanted into the conjunctival sac. Besides its higher secretion quantity per time and the different composition of saliva compared to tear fluid, atrophy of the gland often occurs, and because of these disadvantages it is not a usual procedure. Auto-transplantation of areas of normal conjunctiva from one eye to another is a successful surgical modality, particularly in cases of chemical burns.

3.1.2. Tear Preservation

3.1.2.1. Occlusion of the Tear Drainage System

In advanced cases of KCS, occlusion of the puncta leading into the canaliculi and nasolachrymal sac and duct is able to provide an improvement of both objective and subjective complaints. This is currently the most common non-pharmacological therapy for dry eye disease, it prevents the drainage of natural and artificial tears improving the quantity and quality of the aqueous component.

Patients who underwent punctal occlusion may experience diminished ocular surface sensation and a concomitant decrease in tear production [48], being also possible an increase in toxicity of preservatives present in ocular medications. Besides these disadvantages related with a delay in tear clearance and turnover [49], other complications may be reported such as pruritus, discomfort, deviations and rupture of some plugs, supurative canaliculitis and stenosis. Consequently the decision to occlude all the puncta should not be taken lightly and just after the use of unpreserved tears and lubricants have proven to be insufficient and after a positive result to temporary occlusion with absorbable or removable plugs or inserts.

The easier and most commonly performed techniques are tamponade methods, which occlude the drainage system with a foreign body after a previous anesthesia and punctal dilatation [50]. Non-absorbable tamponade can be achieved by inserting plugs made of silicon, HEMA (hydroxyethylmethacrylate) or Teflon (polytetrafluorethylene) into the canaliculus with the head left protruding from the punctum, being easily removed with forceps or by flushing saline [51]. Inserts made of hydroxypropylcellulose or collagen are absorbable, dissolving slowly at body temperature after insertion into the canaliculus, lasting respectively 18 hours and 2 weeks. These are important to assess the patient's tolerance and avoid future permanent occlusions which may be inadequate in certain cases.

Surgical methods are not usually performed due to the extreme difficulty to reverse them. The exception is the punctum patch, which covers the punctum with autologous conjunctiva and can be easily removed if occlusion results in epiphoria, causing a great deal of discomfort to the patient [52].

When a permanent occlusion is the aim, this usually involves the application of heat, sclerosing or desiccating the lachrymal canaliculi. Thermal methods can be performed by electrically heated probes (cautery), electrodes that coagulate tissues by delivering a high frequency current (diathermy) or argon lasers, being this latter the most flexible method because it can either produce a full or partial occlusion [53].

3.1.2.2. Other Methods of Tear Preservation

Studies have suggested that increased evaporation is one mechanism that produces ocular surface disease associated with dry eyes and some methods of tear preservation act to prevent this evaporation, rather than blocking tear drainage [54]. Moist chambers (watch glass compresses) and tight-fitting goggles (side panels reaching up to the eyebrows) can protect against loss of humidity from the tear film by providing a damp chamber without additional aeration and accumulation of condensation and may, therefore, be useful in more severe cases [55, 56]. Swimming goggles should also be mentioned as protective devices from chlorinated water, worn by patients with KCS. Hyperemizing agents, such as hot eye patches, can be applied over the eyelids for a few minutes, increasing the rate of secretion from the meibomian glands.

The attempt to reverse some of the desiccation seen on the corneal surface, can also be accomplished with bandage soft contact lenses. These water-filled lenses provide a moist covering and exchange some of the fluid with the epithelium, being particularly useful in the dissolution of filamentary keratitis. Besides constituting an irritable foreign body that can worsen the situation, the use of these lenses is associated with the development of bacterial infections and corneal ulcer with endophthalmitis. They must be used in conjunction with artificial tears as they tend to dry out rapidly and are recommended in only a very small number of patients with intractable filamentary keratitis that cannot be managed by any other treatment modality [57].

If no relief occurs upon occlusion of the outgoing lachrymal canaliculi, and for patients with persistent corneal epithelial defects in severe dry eye disease, tarsorrhaphy (i.e., the suturing together a portion of or the entire upper and lower eyelids) can be undertaken. This procedure decreases the exposed surface of the eye, reducing or avoiding the dry out of the pre-corneal tear film between individual blinks. Although quite simple, it shows however the disadvantage of being cosmetically disfigurating [58].

3.1.3. Pharmacological Stimulation of Natural Tears

Small molecular naturally occurring chemicals and some analogs have been identified that stimulate lachrymal gland secretion. This stimulation is able to act only if a sufficient amount of functioning glandular tissue is still available, since no medication is able to stimulate secretion from an atrophied gland. Some drugs, such as mucolytics (bromhexidine and ambroxol), cholinergic agents (carbachol, bethanecol, pilocarpine), or eledoisin, a natural endekapeptide extracted from the salivary glands of the Mediterranean octopus Eledone moschata, have been adopted into therapy [59].

Although with an unknown mechanism of action, the increase in tear secretion produced is doubtless connected with hyperemia due to vasodilation, and theoretically, drugs that can increase cyclic nucleotide (cAMP or cGMP) levels, increase tear secretion [60].

Apart from the fact that the success of this kind of therapy is often questionable, drugs are expensive and the patient may experience a burning sensation when applying them. It is also possible that the stimulation of previously inflamed ocular surface, as in cases of extreme dryness, could deliver pro-inflammatory tears, worsening the disease.

3.1.4. Treatment of the Underlying Causes of Dry Eye Disease

Although the primary mechanism is a qualitative or quantitative defect in the tear film layers, some types of dry eye are caused by immunological or other primary disorders. Inflammatory mediators liberated by the infiltrating T-cells into the lachrymal gland and conjunctiva, such as IFN-γ, and TNF-α cause lachrymal dysfunction, interfere with normal differentiation, and promote apoptosis of lachrymal gland and ocular surface epithelial cells [61, 62]. Increased levels of inflammatory cytokines have also been demonstrated, especially interleukin-6 (IL-6), in the eyes of patients with or without Sjögren's syndrome [27]. Although the correlation of these findings with the lack of hormonal support, chronic irritation and altered innervational mechanisms in some dry eye states are unknown [4, 63], it is predicted that topical anti-inflammatory, immunomodulatory or hormonal agents may be capable of normalizing the disturbed neuro-hormonal reflex between the ocular surface and lachrymal glands. Treatment of any other condition involving conjunctival and corneal surfaces, like a deficit in vitamin A or epidermal growth factor, may complement therapies for dry eye.

3.1.4.1. Cyclosporine A

For the treatment of patients with KCS having primary inflammation of the ocular surface, particularly those who show moderate to severe inflammation, rheumatoid nodules, scleritis and corneal ulcers, immunomodulating agents may be appropriate. Cyclosporine A, largely used to prevent reactions after transplants and in a variety of autoimmune diseases, is an important immunomodulating drug that can also be used in dry eye states.

The efficiency of cyclosporine ophthalmic emulsion for treatment of dry eye was first examined in a randomized, double-masked, placebo-controlled, dose-ranging clinical trial [64]. Although no clear dose-response relationship was seen, cyclosporine 0.05% and 0.1% emulsions provided significant improvements in symptoms, superficial punctate keratitis, and rose bengal staining from baseline. Cyclosporine 0.05% ophthalmic emulsion was approved by the FDA to increase tear production in patients whose tear production is presumed to be suppressed due to ocular inflammation [65].

Many chronic ocular surface disorders share features with dry eye disease, and their responses to immunomodulation therapy with cyclosporine have been evaluated. Because of this, a number of recent studies have examined topical cyclosporine therapy for various ocular surface disorders. In these trials, cyclosporine 0.05% ophthalmic emulsion showed promise for treatment of posterior blepharitis [66], Laser-assisted in situ keratomileusis associated dry eye [67], contact lens intolerance [68], atopic keratoconjunctivitis [69], and herpetic stromal keratitis [70]. Increasingly evidence demonstrates that topical treatment with cyclosporine A prevents T-cell activation and reverses inflammation, improving symptoms and signs of dry eye disease.

3.1.4.2. Topical Corticosteroids

In recent studies, topical corticosteroids have shown promising results for treating dry eye, as they may help increasing goblet cell density and reduce the accumulation of inflammatory cells within ocular surface tissues [71, 72]. Lee et al. reported that ocular surface nerve growth factor (NGF) may play an important role in ocular surface inflammation processes associated with dry eye, since KCS patients showed elevated levels of tear NGF, which decreased by treatment with 0.1% prednisolone [73].

The inflammatory factors are decreased and the integrity of ocular surface is improved after the application of corticosteroid, the nerves of cornea and conjunctiva can be stimulated by blinking more effectively. The reflective secretion becomes normal, then the quality and quantity of tears are also improved. Although corticosteroid can ameliorate the symptoms and signs rapidly, its chronic use for dry eye and for almost any other ocular disease must be restricted, because of severe side effects (e.g., increased infection, ocular hypertension, and cataract formation), being therefore more suitable for acute treatment of dry eye exacerbations.

3.1.4.3. Non-Steroidal Anti-Inflammatory Drugs (NSAIDs)

Topical non-steriodal anti-inflammatory drugs (NSAIDs) are nowadays widely used for the treatment of several ocular conditions, including corneal traumatic and inflammatory diseases and could be considered a good alternative to steroids to avoid the well known complications of corticotherapy in the treatment of patients with chronic diseases.

NSAIDs can be useful in resolving symptoms of ocular discomfort in Sjögren's syndrome patients [74]. A more complete study about the role of these agents in dry eye disease should be therefore undertaken. However, these drugs should be used with caution and under close monitoring, and the treatment should be promptly discontinued if corneal epithelial defects develop or worsen during treatment. The most commonly reported adverse effects are symptoms of stinging and irritation, superficial punctate keratitis, corneal infiltrates and melting [75, 76].

3.1.4.4. Systemic Tetracyclines

Typical bacterial conjunctivitis is caused by the common staphylococcus and diplococcus pneumoniae to the less common organisms of the haemophilus group. Infection is generally in both eyes with the patients experiencing discomfort in the form of grittiness, moderate photophobia and minimal pain. Discharge from the infection causes symptoms of eyelids stuck together on wakening and a "crusty" appearance. Bacterial conjunctivitis responds well to lid hygiene and topical ointments of antibiotics alone or in combination with steroids [77]. In severe cases oral tetracycline and its derivates (e.g., doxycycline) is the treatment of choice, especially in rosacea-associated meibomitis [78].

3.1.4.5. Sexual Hormones

As noted earlier, evidence has strengthened the link between hormonal dysfunction and ocular surface disease, and as androgen and estrogen receptors are widely distributed on the ocular surface and lachrymal gland tissues [79], they represent potential targets for topical application of these hormones as an effective therapy for aqueous-deficient and evaporative dry eye. A topical estradiol-ointment was tested in a clinical trial, proving great potential to improve KCS symptoms [80].

3.1.4.6. Topical Vitamin A

Vitamin A is provided to the corneal epithelium by tears and can exist in three forms, namely, retinol, retinal and retinoic acid, being this latter the most abundant. This nutrient is known to regulate the proliferation and differentiation of corneal epithelial cells and to preserve conjunctival goblet cells. Thus, a lack of vitamin A in the eye may be responsible for xerophthalmia, a keratinisation or formation of a horny layer and drying out of the conjunctiva and cornea, which may produce blindness.

There are serious ocular complications derived from the systemic use of retinoid acid derivates (mainly 13-cis-retinoic acid and isotretinoin), including dry eye signs and symptoms, blepharoconjunctivitis and contact lens intolerance. Bearing this in mind, the indication for therapy with vitamin A is limited to those patients with a loss of goblet cells in very severe dry eye conditions. Usually, vitamin A has been used in the form of a 0.01% ophthalmic ointment, as an adjunct therapy with artificial lubricants in the treatment of eye diseases, such as dry eye and superior limbic keratoconjunctivitis [81, 82]. In 1985 Tseng demonstrated that topical all-trans retinoic acid ointment was effective in the treatment of severe cases of KCS, Stevens-Johnson syndrome, drug-induced pseudopemphigoid, and surgery-induced dry eye, being useful in reversing cellular changes noted in the conjunctiva [83].

3.1.4.7. Topical Autologous Serum

Autologous serum eyedrops have been proposed as a way to deliver essential tear components, e.g., epidermal growth factor, hepatocyte growth factor, fibronectin, neurotrophic growth factor and vitamin A. All of these have shown to play an important role in maintaining ocular surface epithelial milieu and are not included in commercially available artificial tear preparations. Although this kind of treatment is beneficial in cases of persistent epithelial defects [84], superior limbic keratoconjunctivitis [85] and neurotrophic keratopathy [86], because of the nature of study designs and presence of punctum plug occlusion in the patients, its solitary effects were not assessed till recently. A randomized case-control prospective study found significant improvements in tear stability, ocular surface vital staining scores, and pain symptom scores in patients treated with autologous serum eye drops compared with other assigned to non-preserved artificial tears, none of which had punctal occlusion [87]. Autologous serum provides growth factors and vitamins that are useful for an altered ocular surface. However, there are some problems preventing its widespread use in ocular disorders, including risk of contamination, arbitrary dilution, and a current lack of regulations.

3.1.4.8. Omega-6

Recent studies have shown the beneficial effect of oral omega-6 supplementation (γ-linolenic acid and its precursor linoleic acid) in Sjögren's syndrome and dry eye with an inflammatory component [88, 89]. Reduced symptoms of dry eye were reported, as well as an improvement in objective signs such as corneal staining and reduced conjunctival expression of HLA-DR (human leukocyte antigens involved in several autoimmune conditions, disease susceptibility and disease resistance) [90]. Supplementation with linoleic and γ-linoleic acids was shown to increase tear production and reduce dry eye symptoms after photorefractive keratectomy [49].

3.1.4.9. Botulinum Toxin A

Botulinum toxin A, a dichain protein, is one of seven neurotoxins produced by *Clostridium botulinum*. When injected locally, it causes paralysis of the orbicularis oculi muscle by interfering with the release of acetylcholine at neuromuscular junctions. This paralysis acts on the canaliculi inducing a decreased pump function during blink. Because of the reduction of lachrymal drainage after botulinum toxin A injections, this treatment has been suggested for dry eyes [91]. Studies confirmed increased tearing after injections in the eyes of Sjögren's syndrome patients with severe xerophthalmia and blepharospasm [92], and decreased lachrymal drainage after injections in dry eye patients [93]. However, when applied to patients with pathologic hyperlachrymation, a significant reduction of this lachrymation is observed [94]. Further studies are required to assess the clinical value of these injections as an additional treatment for dry eye patients.

3.1.4.10. Acupuncture

Acupuncture is an ancient technique that has shown some benefit in the treatment of Sjögren's syndrome related xerostomia [95] and of KCS [96]. Although acupuncture is not in the common clinical practice of ophthalmologists, their positive effects are attributed to parasympathetic activation not producing any adverse effects. Thus longer observations in a significant number of patients to optimize the technique and further prospective objective measurements of both the tear film and its components should be the subjects of further research.

3.1.4.11. Antiviral Agents

Adenoviral infections are some of the most common external eye infections, causing inflammation of the membrane on the back of the eyelid. Evidence has been accumulated about the associations of viruses with Sjögren's syndrome, such as Epstein-Barr, Human Herpes and Human T lymphotropic virus [97, 98]. Antiretrovirals such as zidovudine, must be tested to assess the tolerance and efficacy in improving dry eye symptoms and signs since they may be beneficial in primary Sjögren's syndrome [99-101]. As new information about novel therapeutic molecules becomes available, designs for clinical trials undoubtedly will undergo further evolution. This is critical to surmount the regulatory barriers to successful development of new, more efficient treatments for patients with dry eye disease.

3.2. Novel Therapeutic Strategies

3.2.1. Polymeric Nanoparticles

Various types of natural and synthetic polymers were used for preparation of nanoparticulate carriers of drugs relevant in dry eye syndrome therapy. The materials and production methods are being extensively reviewed [3, 102]. By selection or further chemical modification of the polymer structure, the characteristics necessary for drug loading and increase of bioavailability in target tissues may be accomplished.

The selection of the material used for production of nanoparticles for ocular delivery should consider the ocular tolerance of the material, and its stability in the tear film i.e. in presence of lysozyme and mucin. Likewise, the material should not interact with mucin of ocular surface to large extent, no significant increase of mucin viscosity should be observed, as increased mucin viscosity may lead to further eye structure damage [103].

Polymers such as poly(D,L-lactic-co-glycolic)acid (PLGA) or poly-ε-caprolactone (PECL) attracted much attention for nanoparticle preparation since these materials are biodegradable [104] and generally biocompatible [102]. Their suitability for ocular delivery has also been shown for several formulations. In fact, no mucosa damage [105] or irritation [106] were observed after PLGA nanoparticles administration in rabbit eyes up to 24 hours by corneal hydration test. With respect to improvement of bioavailability of the drugs in ocular tissues, mucoadhesive polymers are interesting to improve residence time in the eye.

PLGA nanoparticles were proposed for delivery of NSAIDs such as diclofenac sodium salt [106] and flurbiprofen [105]. In this latter case, the drug is available from the nanoparticles in non-dissociated form, in contrast to marketed formulations containing sodium salt. Corneal permeation of flurbiprofen from this system was shown to be superior to aqueous solution or even to a marketed formulation containing a penetration enhancer (e.g., polyvinyl alcohol).

Other NSAIDs have been encapsulated in Eudragit RL and RS, which are copolymers of polyethylacrylate, methyl-methacrylate, and chlorotrimethyl-ammonioethylmethacrylate. Although not showing mucoadhesive properties themselves, these polymers provide a positively charged surface of nanoparticles with a very small diameter, which could enable them to remain onto the ocular surface for the required time to assure efficient drug release [107]. Suspensions of nanoparticles prepared from Eudragit RS and RL were shown non toxic and well tolerated upon administration onto the eye surface [107-109]. Encapsulation of flurbiprofen and ibuprofen led to increased drug concentration in the aqueous humor of the eye despite applying lower concentrations than those in commercially available eye drops. Therefore, these systems were proposed to help maintain miosis during cataract surgery [108, 109]. These systems could also be useful in dry eye syndrome therapy. Nevertheless, formulations aiming to target the anterior eye segments are already reported in the literature.

Cyclosporine A is typically studied as a model drug in various colloidal drug delivery systems. Nanoparticles prepared from e.g. PECL [110] or poly-isobutyl-cyanoacrylate (PIBCA) [111] were examined for the possibility to increase the drug concentration that would permeate the cornea and increase the availability of this peptide for further ocular tissues. Despite various methodologies used to evaluate the drug concentration in the eye, the colloidal carrier systems were clearly more efficient than any oil solution of cyclosporine A. For example, nanocapsules composed of PECL as polymeric shell and medium chain triglycerides as oil core could assure 5 times higher concentration, in comparison to the oily solution, that could be remained within 3 days after administration [110]. An interesting comparison of cyclosporine A nanocapsules, carbopol hydrogel and nanocapsules-loaded hydrogel formulations was assessed by an *ex vivo* study [111]. All of these formulations being superior in effectively of corneal absorption than olive oil solution, the achieved concentrations increased from nanocapsules followed by hydrogel and reaching nanocapsules-loaded hydrogel the highest values. In addition, a slight ocular surface damage was seen for carbopol hydrogel or nanocapsules formulation but not for nanocapsules-loaded hydrogel formulation.

The highest cyclosporine A concentrations were reported from PECL nanoparticles with mucoadhesive coating (hyaluronic acid) and cationic surfactant/preservative (benzalkonium chloride) [112]. The concentrations of cyclosporine A in cornea and conjunctiva were found 6-8 times higher when compared to cyclosporine A administered dissolved in castor oil. Administration of cyclosporine A in hyaluronic acid coated nanoparticles lead to significantly increased uptake of the drug by cornea, especially during the first 4 hours after administration.

In case of treatment of inflammation of the exterior parts of the eye, which is the case of KCS, the increase of drug concentration needs to be carefully considered. It is of high importance to achieve therapeutic concentration of administered drugs in cornea and conjunctiva while not reaching irrelevant tissues and avoiding systemic absorption of the drug. This requires a careful selection of the materials and dosage forms used in dry eye syndrome treatment, so that only the target tissues are exposed to the drug. The nanoparticles not always penetrate the cornea but they rather stay adsorbed on its surface or in the cul-de-sac and act as drug reservoir. Together with the fact the drug release from the carrier is quite slow and continuous; the bioavailability of the drug can be improved.

3.2.1.1. Natural Polymers

Among the polymeric material with the highest relative mucoadhesive properties, hyaluronic acid, sodium alginate and mostly chitosan are investigated for ocular delivery improvement.

Chitosan is a modified (deacetylated) naturally occurring polysaccharide with positive charge. Depending on degree of deacetylation and molecular weight, slight differences in its characteristics are present. Chitosan draw much attention in ocular drug delivery systems design as it shows excellent mucoadhesive properties [113]. These are ascribed to the ability of its amonium groups to bind with sialic acid residues of mucin. Non-modified chitosan is water insoluble at physiological pH, but is capable of swelling [33], which makes it a suitable material for hydrogel and nanoparticle preparation chitosan properties can be further modified by derivatisation of its amino groups. This offers possibility to synthesise wide spectra of chitosan derivates with different solubility conditions and subsequently varying penetration rate. For example, a quaternized derivative N-trimethylchitosan chloride is water-soluble irrespectively of pH, which makes this material a useful transmucosal penetration enhancer [114]. On the other hand, an amphiphilic cholesterol-3-hemisuccinate-chitosan derivate insoluble in neutral pH and self-assembling into particles with size well below 1 µm could be maintained in cornea (78.3%) and conjunctiva (20.1% as measured by γ-scintigraphy of ^{99m}Tc-labeled nanoparticles) without permeating into the posterior segment of the eye [115]. This clearly shows the suitability of Chitosan to design tailor-made systems for reaching the desired part of the eye.

Chitosan nanoparticles can be obtained by simple preparation method – ionic gelation, based on the interaction of the cationic polymer with pentasodium tripolyphosphate [116]. Despite using mild conditions in terms of temperature or pressure, the use of organic solvents is not avoided. Chitosan nanoparticles were intensively tested for their biocompatibility with ocular tissues, with an optimized performance. Almost 100% viability on relevant cell lines was observed (IOBA NHC [117], Chang cells [103]), no irritation or damage in the outer ocular tissues after *in vivo* testing. De Campos et al. evaluated the stability of chitosan nanoparticles in conditions similar to those physiological of eye surface [103]. Again, the suitability of these systems was confirmed, as the nanoparticles did not suffer any degradation in presence of lysozyme or mucin. Also, mucin viscosity was not affected by the presence of such polysaccharide-based systems. The potential of chitosan in ocular drug delivery, illustrated by many nanoparticle or nanocapsules formulations or colloidal carriers coatings, was recently reviewed by Paolicelli et al. [33].

Cyclosporine A-loaded chitosan nanoparticles were instilled in eye rabbits following bioavailability assessment in conjunctiva and cornea, in comparison to a cyclosporine solution in chitosan or water [118]. Peptide concentration was significantly higher after administration of nanoparticles than of the solutions. The therapeutic dose could be maintained in conjunctiva and cornea up to 48 hours. These chitosan nanoparticles were shown to accumulate in the external ocular tissues, and to remain on the ocular surface. It was therefore anticipated that chitosan nanoparticles have higher affinity to conjunctiva than cornea [103]. In case of cyclosporine A, small quantities of drug were detected in systemic circulation, however, in such a concentration that is not expected to cause any side effects [118]. With regard to concentrations reached within the eye (i.e., iris/ciliary body and aqueous humour), blood and plasma, clearly highest concentration could be found in external ocular tissues, intraocular concentrations of the drug was not enhanced. Considering ocular surface diseases, such as the KCS, this characteristic make non-modified chitosan a very promising material for drug delivery systems design.

Indomethacin-loaded chitosan nanoparticles were also tested for ocular wound healing purposes [34]. Upon application on healthy eye, normal histological image of cornea was obtained. For this purpose, a chitosan nanoemulsion was favoured over chitosan nanoparticles.

3.2.1.2. Polymeric Coating of Various Carrier Systems

The effectiveness of colloidal carriers on the eye strongly depends on their surface characteristics. As shown by various research groups, presence and type of the coating of the colloidal carriers are governing its ability to permeate through cornea. A comparison between polyethylene glycol (PEG)-coated and chitosan-coated PECL nanocapsules clearly showed that the surface characteristics influence the fate of the nanoparticles in the eye. While PEG-coated nanocapsules could proceed through the cornea by transcellular pathway, chitosan coated particles could enter the corneal cells, but were maintain within them [119]. By selecting the surface characteristics of the colloidal carrier, it can be targeted to the particular part of the eye. Chitosan has been used as coating of various colloidal carriers intended for ocular drug delivery. These include nanoparticles prepared from various polymers [120], lipid nanoparticles [121] or liposomes [122, 123]. The combination of chitosan with phospholipids seems to be in particular useful in ocular drug delivery. The complexes prepared from these materials, either chitosan-coated liposomes [124] or chitosan nanoparticles with a phospholipid shell [122], could penetrate through corneal tissues easily. Depending on composition, the extent of the permeation could be controlled. A hyaluronic acid coating may also be used to enhance cyclosporine A concentration in corneal tissues reported after administration of nanoparticles [112].

3.2.2. Solid Lipid Nanoparticles

Colloidal carriers based on lipids offer the advantage of use of naturally occurring or very similar material, which is presumed to be well tolerated and non toxic. These characteristics need however to be shown for every type of material and stabilizing agent used for the manufacture. Since ophthalmic emulsions have already reached the market, one might antecipate that other lipid-based drug delivery systems applications will be seen in near future.

Lipid nanoparticles were developed after polymeric nanoparticles on the concept of replacing the oil phase of an emulsion by a solid lipid and thus obtaining particles with small size (50-1000 nm) that are solid at room temperature. Lipid nanoparticles already tested for ocular delivery include solid lipid nanoparticles (SLN), nanostructured lipid carriers (NLC). The production methods and drug incorporation models are reviewed elsewhere [125].

Suitability of lipid nanoparticles for ocular drug delivery was first shown by Cavalli *et al.* who reported a tobramycin-loaded SLN formulation [126]. Already in this study, prolonged pre-corneal residence times were observed when compared to an aqueous solution of fluorescamine, and higher bioavailability of the incorporated drug than from a marketed aqueous solution was achieved. With regards to KCS, NSAIDs and cyclosporine A formulations were also reported.

Ibuprofen-loaded NLC could be used to improve ocular bioavailability, which could be further enhanced by stearylamine incorporation to obtain a positive surface charge. Thus the pre-corneal retention times could be prolonged [127]. Diclofenac sodium salt was encapsulated SLN composed of a mixture of lipid from goat fat plated with a phospholipid [128]. The coating was found to be important factor influencing both the release of diclofenac from the particles, as well as its penetration through cornea construct. The phospholipid coating was the prerequisite of controlled release and higher permeation rate through the cornea [129].

Several research groups developed SLN formulations to deliver cyclosporine A. As this peptide is poorly soluble in water, a lipid based system may be a successful solution for its formulation. Formulations with particle size less than 500 nm and stability over 6 months were reported [130], and, as expected, typically high loading capacities (over 90%) were achieved [131, 132]. Both blank and cyclosporine-loaded SLN were biocompatible with rabbit corneal epithelium (RCE) cells, maintaining the percentage of living cells comparable with those cultivated with growth medium [131].

Penetration or permeation of cyclosporine A suspension into RCE cells or excised corneal tissues could not be observed in several reports [121, 131], but cyclosporine could be detected within the cells [121] and found to permeate the corneal tissues [121, 131] after being delivered by SLN. However, Gokce *et al.* did not find the differences between the permeation of cyclosporine A suspension and protein-loaded SLN significantly [131]. An *in vivo* study showed that cyclosporine administered in SLN could eventually reach the vitreous body of the eye and could be detected 48 hours after administration [133].

The pre-corneal residence time of SLN or NLC formulations could be further improved by inducing positive surface charge e.g. by stearylamine [130, 134], or by mucoadhesive coating cysteine-PEG stearate coating [135]. To improve the ability to permeate the corneal tissue, nanoparticles prepared from solid lipid and chitosan mixtures were proposed [121]. Indeed, in cell culture these formulations have proven to be more efficient to enhance cyclosporine A penetration into epithelial cells. All of these reports show the potential of lipid nanoparticles to be used in ocular therapy for cyclosporine.

Considering the practical point of view, the lipid nanoparticle formulations could be sterilized either by autoclaving [130, 131] or by freeze-drying [136] without compromising the colloidal nature of the formulations. The methods used in preparation of the referred formulations are generally simple and do should be applicable in large scale production as well. If low wt% of lipid is used in the formulation, it remains liquid and slightly opalescent, which should not cause much inconvenience upon ocular administration. Despite these promising results, there are still only a few reports on SLN or NLC for ocular drug delivery. Practical use of these formulations can be considered only after conveying more detailed studies.

3.2.3. Liposomes

Liposomes are drug delivery systems suitable for delivery of both hydrophilic and lipophilic drugs, feasible for various administration routes [137]. Extensive testing of liposomes application in ophthalmology revealed their suitability in terms of sufficient bioavailability improvement of drugs relevant in ocular diseases treatment and acceptable toxicological profile [138]. The mechanisms of bioavailability improvement of drugs administered in liposomes may include their adherence to the ocular surface, as well as the optimal rate of drug release. Prolonged residence times on corneal surface where observed with liposomes with positive surface charge.

Examples of ocular bioavailability improvements by liposome encapsulation include NSAIDs [139], and immunosupressives, such as the sirolimus or rapamycin, which was found in therapeutic concentrations throughout the eye when administered in liposomes [140]. Immunosuppressive peptides, antibiotics, and NSAIDs, are often formulated in different colloidal carriers, which may be superior to liposomes in terms of stability upon administration, also long term storage stability and manufacture costs. What makes liposomes in particular relevant in KCS therapy is the composition of natural (or similar to natural) amphiphilic phospholipids. There are strong evidences that evaporative dry eye needs treatment focused on the lipid layer of the tear film. Aqueous tear supplements are not sufficient in these cases, as well as there might be no need for administration of immunosuppressives. Although artificial tears and ophthalmic gels with triglyceride content are commercially available and do bring relief in this type of KCS, liposomal formulations were proposed. Currently, there are two liposome-containing over-the-counter products available on the market (TearsAgain Liposome Spray™, Optima Pharmaceutical GmbH and Clarymist™). Both are administered on closed eyelids. A few reports from clinical studies of these formulations indicate their significantly superior clinical benefits over triglyceride containing eye gel [141], or aqueous artificial tears eye drops [142], or sprays [143] presented in some controlled parameters. Improvements were reported in particular in eyelid edge inflammation. These data hint that phospholipids administered in form of colloidal carriers might be more beneficial than in form of solution or gel. However, a direct proof of the proposed mechanism of action (improvement of tear film stability) is still missing. Also, the price of these products is considerably higher than that of any conventional ophthalmic formulation.

Chapter IV

Conclusions and Future Trends

The research and development of advanced drug delivery systems may bring additional advantages in the management of KCS. The materials and formulations summarized here show potential of improving the bioavailability of the drugs relevant in KCS management. Since only a few of these systems reached the pharmaceutical market in any administration route (Liposomes in i.v., dermal and ocular; NLC in dermal), the prior concern of these systems would be their actual safety upon administration in human eye. Various methods were used to assess the safety of the proposed systems making the comparison of the different types of colloidal carrier unclear; however, the most of these results are positive in terms of sufficient safety.

Table 1 gives an overview of the drug incorporated in different colloidal carriers and the advantages reported from their testing. The formulations of NSAIDs group generally achieved longer residence time onto the ocular surface, and can deliver also water insoluble drugs such as flurbiprofen or diclofenac in their non-dissociated form. Except from chitosan-coated formulations, the NSAIDs were loaded into material which does not show much pronounced mucoadhesive properties. The improved pre-corneal residence times could be attributed to the positive charge the nanoparticles had, and simply to the colloidal size of these particles, assuring slightly adhesive properties.

Table 1. Examples of drugs entrapped into colloidal carriers based on polymeric, polyssacharide or lipid materials, for ocular administration

Drug	Formulation	Improvements	Reference
Cyclosporine-A	PIBCA NS PIBCA NS incorporated in Carbopol hydrogel	Higher effectiveness in corneal absorption of drug as compared to olive oil solution; limited damage of corneal tissue (NS hydrogel)	[111]
	PECL NP	Increase in AUC, therapeutic concentrations maintained during 3 days	[110]
	Hyaluronic acid coated PECL NS	6-8 times higher corneal levels than from castor oil emulsion, higher corneal uptake of the drug in first 4 hours after administration	[145]
	Chitosan NP	Therapeutic dose maintained for 24 hours in conjunctiva; 48 hours in cornea	[118]
	SLN	Enhanced permeation and penetration through RCE cells and corneal construct, no ocular irritation nor corneal damage	[130-132, 135, 146]
	Thiolated PEG-coated NLC	Enhanced pre-corneal retention time, controlled release over 12 hours	[135]
Diclofenac	PLGA NP	No irritation up to 24 hours post-administration (Draize test)	[106]
	Eudragit RS NP		[147]
	SLN	Enhanced corneal permeation, non-dissociated drug available	[128, 148]
Ibuprofen	Eudragit RS 100 NP	Therapeutic effect achieved with lower administered concentration	[108, 149]
	Eudragit RL 100 NP		[150]
	NLC	Enhanced pre-corneal retention time	[127]
Flurbiprofen	Eudragit RS RL NP	Higher drug concentration in the aqueous humour achieved in comparison with eye drops, non-dissociated drug available, no corneal damage	[109]
	PLGA NP	Corneal penetration superior to drug buffer solution or drug solution containing PVA	[105, 151]

Drug	Formulation	Improvements	Reference
Indomethacin	Chitosan-coated emulsion		[152]
	Chitosan NE, NPs	NE: significantly higher concentrations in aqueous humour first hour post-administration	[34]
	Chitosan NC	Increased corneal transport	[153]
Piroxicam	Eudragit RS 100	Anti-inflammatory effect observed up to 24 hours	[154]

AUC, area under the curve; NS, nanospheres; NC, nanocapsules; NP, nanoparticles; SLN, solid lipid nanoparticles; NLC, nanostructured lipid carriers, PECL, poly-ε-caprolactone; PEG, polyethylenglycol; PIBCA, poly-isobutyl-cyanoacrylate; PLGA, poly(lactic-co-glycolic)acid; PVA, polyvinyl alcohol; RCE, Rabbit corneal epithelium.

Also cyclosporine A concentration improvements could be achieved using different materials. The highest concentrations reported in the research literature were obtained when using colloidal carriers with mucoadhesive coatings, however, non-adhesive material based carriers could also produce promising results. Cyclosporine A was shown to have the ability to accumulate in cornea and conjunctiva which may act as drug reservoir and release it over extended period of time [144], therefore a high residence time onto the ocular surface, maintained for sufficient time seem to be the most important factor for a successful formulation. Again, the small size gives advantage itself, associated with a positive surface charge might ensure the contact with the ocular surface. As the mucin content may vary drastically in KCS conditions, mucoadhesiveness of the material itself may not be sufficient to enable the drug to stay on the ocular surface for a sufficient time. Therefore, the advantages that colloidal carriers may bring is their bioavailability improvement by enhanced drug permeation into the eye and improved residence time on the ocular surface, which can be assured by adhesiveness, a feature that colloidal carriers typically have, stressed by positive surface charge of the carriers.

References

[1] Holly FJ, Lemp MA: Tear physiology and dry eyes. *Surv. Ophthalmol.* 1977, 22:69-87.

[2] Ali Y, Lehmussaari K: Industrial perspective in ocular drug delivery. *Adv. Drug Deliv. Rev.* 2006, 58:1258-1268.

[3] Nagarwal RC, Kant S, Singh PN, Maiti P, Pandit JK: Polymeric nanoparticulate system: A potential approach for ocular drug delivery. *Journal of Controlled Release.* 2009, 136:2-13.

[4] Stern ME, Beuerman RW, Fox RI, Gao J, Mircheff AK, Pflugfelder SC: A unified theory of the role of the ocular surface in dry eye. *Adv. Exp. Med. Biol.* 1998, 438:643-651.

[5] Niederkorn JY, Stern ME, Pflugfelder SC, De Paiva CS, Corrales RM, Gao J, Siemasko K: Desiccating stress induces T cell-mediated Sjogren's Syndrome-like lacrimal keratoconjunctivitis. *J. Immunol* .2006, 176:3950-3957.

[6] Stern ME, Gao J, Siemasko KF, Beuerman RW, Pflugfelder SC: The role of the lacrimal functional unit in the pathophysiology of dry eye. *Exp. Eye Res.* 2004, 78:409-416.

[7] Nakamori K, Odawara M, Nakajima T, Mizutani T, Tsubota K: Blinking is controlled primarily by ocular surface conditions. *Am. J. Ophthalmol.* 1997, 124:24-30.

[8] Lemp MA, Marquardt R: *The dry eye: A comprehensive guide.* Springer-Verlag (Berlin, New York); 1992.

[9] Kobayashi TK, Tsubota K, Takamura E, Sawa M, Ohashi Y, Usui M: Effect of retinol palmitate as a treatment for dry eye: a cytological evaluation. *Ophthalmologica.* 1997, 211:358-361.

[10] Hatchell DL, Sommer A: Detection of Ocular Surface Abnormalities in Experimental Vitamin A Deficiency. *Arch. Ophthalmol.* 1984, 102:1389-1393.
[11] Brignole F, Pisella PJ, Goldschild M, De Saint Jean M, Goguel A, Baudouin C: Flow cytometric analysis of inflammatory markers in conjunctival epithelial cells of patients with dry eyes. *Invest. Ophthalmol. Vis. Sci.* 2000, 41:1356-1363.
[12] Jones D, Monroy D, Ji Z, Atherton S, Pflugfelder S: Sjogren's syndrome: cytokine and Epstein-Barr viral gene expression within the conjunctival epithelium. *Invest. Ophthalmol. Vis. Sci.* 1994, 35:3493-3504.
[13] Pflugfelder SC, Solomon A, Dursun D: Dry eye and delayed tear clearance: 'a call to arms'. *Adv. Exp. Med. Biol.* 2002, 506:739-743.
[14] Tsubota K, Goto E, Fujita H, Ono M, Inoue H, Saito I, Shimmura S: Treatment of dry eye by autologous serum application in Sjogren's syndrome. *Br. J. Ophthalmol.* 1999, 83:390-395.
[15] Vivino FB, Katz WA: jögren's syndrome: Clinical picture and diagnostic tests. *Journal of Musculoskeletal Medicine.* 1995, 12:40-52.
[16] Foster CS, Rice BA, Dutt JE: Immunopathology of atopic keratoconjunctivitis. *Ophthalmology.* 1991, 98:1190-1196.
[17] Metz D, P., Hingorani M, Calder V, L., Buckley R, J., Lightman S, L.: T-cell cytokines in chronic allergic eye disease. *J. Allergy Clin. Immunol.* 1997, 100:817-824.
[18] Vermeulen A, D. M, D. P: Commentary to the Article--Low Levels of Sex Hormone-Binding Globulin and Testosterone Are Associated with Smaller, Denser Low Density Lipoproteins in Normoglycemic Menc. *J. Clin. Endocrinol. Metab.* 1998, 83:1822a-.
[19] Warren DW: Hormonal Influences on the Lacrimal Gland. *Int. Ophthalmol. Clin.* 1994, 34:19-25.
[20] Sullivan DA, Schaumberg DA, Suzuki T, Schirra F, Liu M, Richards S, Sullivan RM, Dana MR, Sullivan BD: Sex steroids, meibomian gland dysfunction and evaporative dry eye in Sj ogren's syndrome. *Lupus.* 2002, 11:667-.
[21] Sullivan DA, Sullivan BD, Evans JE, Schirra F, Yamagami H, Liu M, Richards SM, Suzuki T, Schaumberg DA, Sullivan RM, Dana MR: Androgen deficiency, meibomian gland dysfunction, and evaporative dry eye. *Am. N.Y. Acad. Sci.* 2002, 966.
[22] Richardson JD, Vasko MR: Cellular Mechanisms of Neurogenic Inflammation. *J. Pharmacol. Exp. Ther.* 2002, 302:839-845.

[23] Nelson JD, Havener VR, Cameron JD: Cellulose Acetate Impressions of the Ocular Surface: Dry Eye States. *Arch. Ophthalmol.* 1983, 101:1869-1872.
[24] Tseng SC, Hirst LW, Maumenee AE, Kenyon KR, Sun TT, Green WR: Possible mechanisms for the loss of goblet cells in mucin-deficient disorders. *Ophthalmology.* 1984, 91:545-552.
[25] Driver P, J. , Lemp M, A. : Meibomian gland dysfunction. *Surv. Ophthalmol.* 1996, 40:343-367.
[26] Shimazaki J, Sakata M, K. T: Ocular surface changes and discomfort in patients with meibomian gland dysfunction. *Arch. Ophthalmol.* 1995, 113:1266-1270.
[27] Pflugfelder SC, Tseng SC, Sanabria O, Kell HOD, Garcia CG, Felix C, Feuer W, Reis BL: Evaluation of subjective assessments and objective diagnostic tests for diagnosing tear-film disorders known to cause ocular irritation. *Cornea.* 1998, 17:38 -56.
[28] Asbell PA: Increasing importance of dry eye syndrome and the ideal artificial tear: consensus views from a roundtable discussion*. *Current Medical Research and Opinion.* 2006, 22:2149-2157.
[29] Bron AJ, Daubas P, Siou-Mermet R, Trinquand C: Comparison of the efficacy and safety of two eye gels in the treatment of dry eyes: Lacrinorm and Viscotears. *Eye.* 1998, 12 (Pt 5):839-847.
[30] Bron AJ, Tiffany JM, Embleton J: Topical delivery of microvolumes using a forced-flow system (Optidyne). In *Lacrimal Gland, Tear Film and Dry Eye Syndromes. Volume* Vol. 2. Edited by (Ed.) SDA. New York: Plenum; 1998
[31] Oechsner M, Keipert S: Polyacrylic acid/polyvinylpyrrolidone bipolymeric systems. I. Rheological and mucoadhesive properties of formulations potentially useful for the treatment of dry-eye-syndrome. *Eur. J. Pharm. Biopharm.* 1999, 47:113-118.
[32] Barbu E, Verestiuc L, Iancu M, Jatariu A, Lungu A, Tsibouklis J: Hybrid polymeric hydrogels for ocular drug delivery: nanoparticulate systems from copolymers of acrylic acid-functionalized chitosan and N-isopropylacrylamide or 2-hydroxyethyl methacrylate. *Nanotechnology.* 2009, 20:225108.
[33] Paolicelli P, de la Fuente M, Sanchez A, Seijo B, Alonso MJ: Chitosan nanoparticles for drug delivery to the eye. *Expert. Opin. Drug Deliv.* 2009, 6:239-253.

[34] Badawi AA, El-Laithy HM, El Qidra RK, El Mofty H, El dally M: Chitosan based nanocarriers for indomethacin ocular delivery. *Arch. Pharm. Res.* 2008, 31:1040-1049.
[35] Lemp MA: Dry eye syndromes: treatment and clinical trials. *Adv. Exp. Med. Biol.* 1994, 350:553-559.
[36] Lemp MA: Management of the dry-eye patient. *Int. Ophthalmol. Clin.* 1994, 34:101-113.
[37] Marchese A, Bozzolasco M, Gualco L, Schito GC, Debbia EA: Evaluation of spontaneous contamination of ocular medications. *Chemotherapy.* 2001, 47:304-308.
[38] Murube J, Murube A, Zhuo C: Classification of artificial tears. II: Additives and commercial formulas. *Adv. Exp. Med. Biol.* 1998, 438:705-715.
[39] Murube J, Paterson A, Murube E: Classification of artificial tears. I: Composition and properties. *Adv. Exp. Med. Biol.* 1998, 438:693-704.
[40] Tripathi BJ, Tripathi RC: Cytotoxic effects of benzalkonium chloride and chlorobutanol on human corneal epithelial cells in vitro. *Lens. Eye Toxic Res.* 1989, 6:395-403.
[41] Murube J: Tear osmolarity. *Ocul. Surf.* 2006, 4:62-73.
[42] Gilbard JP: Human tear film electrolyte concentrations in health and dry-eye disease. *Int. Ophthalmol. Clin.* 1994, 34:27-36.
[43] Gilbard JP, Rossi SR: Changes in tear ion concentrations in dry-eye disorders. *Adv. Exp. Med. Biol.* 1994, 350:529-533.
[44] Ubels JL, McCartney MD, Lantz WK, Beaird J, Dayalan A, Edelhauser HF: Effects of preservative-free artificial tear solutions on corneal epithelial structure and function. *Arch. Ophthalmol.* 1995, 113:371-378.
[45] Wander AH, Koffler BH: Extending the duration of tear film protection in dry eye syndrome: review and retrospective case series study of the hydroxypropyl cellulose ophthalmic insert. *Ocul. Surf.* 2009, 7:154-162.
[46] Diestelhorst M, Grunthal S, Suverkrup R: Dry Drops: a new preservative-free drug delivery system. *Graefes Arch. Clin. Exp. Ophthalmol.* 1999, 237:394-398.
[47] Geerling G, Sieg P, Bastian GO, Laqua H: Transplantation of the autologous submandibular gland for most severe cases of keratoconjunctivitis sicca. *Ophthalmology.* 1998, 105:327-335.
[48] Yen MT, Pflugfelder SC, Feuer WJ: The effect of punctal occlusion on tear production, tear clearance, and ocular surface sensation in normal subjects. *Am. J. Ophthalmol.* 2001, 131:314-323.

[49] Macrì A, Giuffrida S, Amico V, Iester M, Traverso CE: Effect of linoleic acid and gamma-linolenic acid on tear production, tear clearance and on the ocular surface after photorefractive keratectomy. *Greafes Arch. Clin. Exp. Ophthalmol.* 2003, 241:561-566.
[50] Redmond JW: Punctal occlusion with collagen implants. *Ophthalmic Surg.* 1992, 23:642.
[51] Willis RM, Folberg R, Krachmer JH, Holland EJ: The treatment of aqueous-deficient dry eye with removable punctal plugs. A clinical and impression-cytologic study. *Ophthalmology.* 1987, 94:514-518.
[52] Murube J: Surgical treatment of dry eye. *Orbit* 2003, 22:203-232.
[53] Benson DR, Hemmady PB, Snyder RW: Efficacy of laser punctal occlusion. *Ophthalmology.* 1992, 99:618-621.
[54] Rolando M, Refojo MF: Tear evaporimeter for measuring water evaporation rate from the tear film under controlled conditions in humans. *Exp. Eye Res.* 1983, 36:25-33.
[55] Tsubota K, Yamada M, Urayama K: Spectacle side panels and moist inserts for the treatment of dry-eye patients. *Cornea.* 1994, 13:197-201.
[56] Tsubota K: New approaches to dry-eye therapy. *Int. Ophthalmol. Clin.* 1994, 34:115-128.
[57] Farris RL: Contact lenses and the dry eye. *Int. Ophthalmol. Clin.* 1994, 34:129-136.
[58] Stamler JF, Tse DT: A simple and reliable technique for permanent lateral tarsorrhaphy. *Arch. Ophthalmol.* 1990, 108:125-127.
[59] Calonge M: The treatment of dry eye. *Surv. Ophthalmol.* 2001, 45 Suppl 2:S227-239.
[60] Gilbard JP, Rossi SR, Heyda KG, Dartt DA: Stimulation of tear secretion by topical agents that increase cyclic nucleotide levels. *Invest. Ophthalmol. Vis. Sci.* 1990, 31:1381-1388.
[61] Pflugfelder SC, Solomon A, Stern ME: The Diagnosis and Management of Dry Eye: A Twenty-five-Year Review. *Cornea.* 2000, 19:644-649.
[62] Smith RE: The Tear Film Complex: Pathogenesis and Emerging Therapies for Dry Eyes. *Cornea.* 2005, 24:1-7.
[63] Stern ME, Beuerman RW, Fox RI, Gao J, Mircheff AK, Pflugfelder SC: The pathology of dry eye: the interaction between the ocular surface and lacrimal glands. *Cornea.* 1998, 17:584-589.
[64] Stevenson D, Tauber J, Reis BL: Efficacy and safety of cyclosporin a ophthalmic emulsion in the treatment of moderate-to-severe dry eye disease - A dose-ranging, randomized trial. *Ophthalmology.* 2000, 107:967-974.

[65] Sall K, Stevenson OD, Mundorf T, K., Reis B, L. : Two multicenter, randomized studies of the efficacy and safety of cyclosporine ophthalmic emulsion in moderate to severe dry eye disease. *Ophthalmology.* 2000, 107:631-639.
[66] Perry HD, Doshi-Carnevale S, Donnenfeld ED, Solomon Re, Biser SA, Bloom AH: Efficacy of Commercially Available Topical Cyclosporine A 0.05% in the Treatment of Meibomian Gland Dysfunction. *Cornea.* 2006, 25:171-175.
[67] Salib G, M., McDonald M, B., Smolek M: Safety and efficacy of cyclosporine 0.05% drops versus unpreserved artificial tears in dry-eye patients having laser in situ keratomileusis. *J. Cataract Refract. Surg.* 2006, 32:772-778.
[68] Hom MM: Use of Cyclosporine 0.05% Ophthalmic Emulsion for Contact Lens-Intolerant Patients. *Eye Contact Lens.* 2006, 32:109-111.
[69] Akpek EK, Dart JK, Watson S, Christen W, Dursun D, Yoo S, P. T, Schein OD, Gottsch JD: A randomized trial of topical cyclosporin 0.05% in topical steroid-resistant atopic keratoconjunctivitis. *Ophthalmology.* 2004, 111:476-482.
[70] Rao S, N.: Treatment of Herpes Simplex Virus Stromal Keratitis Unresponsive to Topical Prednisolone 1% With Topical Cyclosporine 0.05%. *Am. J. Ophthalmol.* 2006, 141:771-772.
[71] Avunduk AM, Avunduk MC, Varnell ED, Kaufman HE: The comparison of efficacies of topical corticosteroids and nonsteroidal anti-inflammatory drops on dry eye patients: a clinical and immunocytochemical study. *Am. J. Ophthalmol.* 2003, 136:593-602.
[72] Pflugfelder SC, Maskin SL, Anderson B, Chodosh J, Holland EJ, d, e Palva CS, Bartels SP, Micuda T, Proskin HE, Vogel R: A randomized, double-masked, placebo-controlled, multicenter comparison of loteprednol etabonate ophthalmic suspension, 0.5%, and placebo for treatment of keratoconjunctivitis sicca in patients with delayed tear clearance. *Am. J. Ophthalmol.* 2004, 138:444-457.
[73] Lee HK, Ryu IH, Seo KY, Hong S, Kim HC, Kim EK: Topical 0.1% Prednisolone Lowers Nerve Growth Factor Expression in Keratoconjunctivitis Sicca Patients. *Ophthalmology.* 2006, 113:198-205.
[74] Avisar R, Robinson A, Appel I, Yassur Y, Weinberger D: Diclofenac sodium, 0.1% (Voltaren Ophtha), versus sodium chloride, 5%, in the treatment of filamentary keratitis. *Cornea.* 2000, 19:145-147.

[75] Guidera A, C. , Luchs J, I., Udell I, J. : Keratitis, ulceration, and perforation associated with topical nonsteroidal anti-inflammatory drugs. *Ophthalmology.* 2001, 108:936-944.

[76] Hsu J, K. W., Johnston WT, Read R, W., McDonnell P, J. , Pangalinan R, Rao N, Smith R, E. : Histopathology of corneal melting associated with diclofenac use after refractive surgery. *J. Cataract Refract. Surg.* 2003, 29:250-256.

[77] Dougherty JM, McCulley JP, Silvany RE, Meyer DR: The role of tetracycline in chronic blepharitis. Inhibition of lipase production in staphylococci. *Invest. Ophthalmol. Vis. Sci.* 1991, 32:2970-2975.

[78] Cetinkaya A, Akova YA: Pediatric ocular acne rosacea: long-term treatment with systemic antibiotics. *Am. J. Ophthalmol.* 2006, 142:816-821.

[79] Esmaeli B, Harvey JT, Hewlett B: Immunohistochemical evidence for estrogen receptors in meibomian glands. *Ophthalmology.* 2000, 107:180-184.

[80] Akramian J, Wedrich A, Nepp J, Sator M: Estrogen therapy in keratoconjunctivitis sicca. *Adv. Exp. Med. Biol.* 1998, 438:1005-1009.

[81] Ohashi Y, Watanabe H, Kinoshita S, Hosotani H, Umemoto M, R. M: Vitamin A eye drops for superior limbic keratoconjunctivitis. *Am. J. Ophthalmol.* 1988, 105:523-527.

[82] Selek H, Unlü N, Orhan M, M. I: Evaluation of retinoic acid ophthalmic emulsion in dry eye. *Eur. J. Ophthalmol.* 2000, 10:121-127.

[83] Tseng S: Topical retinoid treatment for dry eye disorders. *Trans. Ophthalmol. Soc. U.K.* 1985, 104:489-495.

[84] Tsubota K, Shimazaki J: Surgical treatment of children blinded by Stevens-Johnson syndrome. *Am. J. Ophthalmol.* 1999, 128:573-581.

[85] Goto E, Shimmura S, Shimazaki J, Tsubota K: Treatment of Superior Limbic Keratoconjunctivitis by Application of Autologous Serum. *Cornea.* 2001, 20:807-810.

[86] Matsumoto Y, Dogru M, Goto E, Ohashi Y, Kojima T, Ishida R, Tsubota K: Autologous serum application in the treatment of neurotrophic keratopathy. *Ophthalmology.* 2004, 111:1115-1120.

[87] Kojima T, Ishida R, Dogru M, Goto E., Matsumoto Y, Kaido M, Tsubota K: The effect of autologous serum eyedrops in the treatment of severe dry eye disease: A prospective randomized case-control study. *Am. J. Ophthalmol.* 2005, 139:242-246.

[88] Aragona P, Bucolo C, Spinella R, Giuffrida S, Ferreri G: Systemic Omega-6 Essential Fatty Acid Treatment and PGE1 Tear Content in

Sjogren's Syndrome Patients. *Invest. Ophthalmol. Vis. Sci.* 2005, 46:4474-4479.

[89] Barabino S, Rolando M, Camicione P, Ravera G, Zanardi S, Giuffrida S, Calabria G: Systemic Linoleic and [gamma]-Linolenic Acid Therapy in Dry Eye Syndrome With an Inflammatory Component. *Cornea.* 2003, 22:97-101.

[90] Tsubota K, Fujihara T, Saito K, Takeuchi T: Conjunctival epithelium expression of HLA-DR in dry eye patients. *Ophthalmologica.* 1999, 213:16-19.

[91] Sahlin S, Chen E: Evaluation of the lacrimal drainage function by the drop test. *Am. J. Ophthalmol.* 1996, 122:701-708.

[92] Spiera H, Asbell PA, Simpson DM: Botulinum toxin increases tearing in patients with Sjogren's syndrome: a preliminary report. *J. Rheumatol.* 1997, 24:1842-1843.

[93] Sahlin S, Chen E, Kaugesaar T, Almqvist H, Kjellberg K, Lennerstrand G: Effect of eyelid botulinum toxin injection on lacrimal drainage. *Am. J. Ophthalmol.* 2000, 129:481-486.

[94] Riemann R, Pfennigsdorf S, Riemann E, Naumann M: Successful treatment of crocodile tears by injection of botulinum toxin into the lacrimal gland: a case report. *Ophthalmology.* 1999, 106:2322-2324.

[95] Blom M, Kopp S, Lundeberg T: Prognostic value of the pilocarpine test to identify patients who may obtain long-term relief from xerostomia by acupuncture treatment. *Arch. Otolaryngol. Head Neck Surg.* 1999, 125:561-566.

[96] Nepp J, Derbolav A, Haslinger-Akramian J, Mudrich C, Schauersberger J, Wedrich A: [Effect of acupuncture in keratoconjunctivitis sicca]. *Klin. Monatsbl. Augenheilkd.* 1999, 215:228-232.

[97] Tsubota K, Fujishima H, Toda I, Katagiri S, Kawashima Y, Saito I: Increased levels of Epstein-Barr virus DNA in lacrimal glands of Sjogren's syndrome patients. *Acta Ophthalmol. Scand.* 1995, 73:425-430.

[98] Willoughby CE, Baker K, Kaye SB, Carey P, O'Donnell N, Field A, Longman L, Bucknall R, Hart CA: Epstein-Barr virus (types 1 and 2) in the tear film in Sjogren's syndrome and HIV infection. *J. Med. Virol.* 2002, 68:378-383.

[99] Pot C, Chizzolini C, Vokatch N, Tiercy JM, Ribi C, Landis T, Perren F: Combined antiviral-immunosuppressive treatment in human T-lymphotrophic virus 1-Sjogren-associated myelopathy. *Arch. Neurol.* 2006, 63:1318-1320.

[100] Steinfeld S, Simonart T: New approaches to the treatment of Sjogren's syndrome: soon beyond symptomatic relief? *Dermatology.* 2003, 207:6-9.
[101] Steinfeld SD, Demols P, Van Vooren JP, Cogan E, Appelboom T: Zidovudine in primary Sjogren's syndrome. *Rheumatology. (Oxford)* 1999, 38:814-817.
[102] Moghimi SM, Vega E, Garcia ML, Al-Hanbali OAR, Rutt KJ: Polymeric nanoparticles as drug carriers and controlled release implant devices. In *Nanoparticulates as drug carriers.* Edited by Torchilin VP. London: Imperial College Press; 2006: 29-42
[103] de Campos A, Diebold Y, Carvalho E, Sánchez A, José Alonso M: Chitosan Nanoparticles as New Ocular Drug Delivery Systems: in Vitro Stability, in Vivo Fate, and Cellular Toxicity. *Pharm. Res.* 2004, 21:803-810.
[104] Deshpande A, Heller J, Gurny R: Bioerodible polymers for ocular delivery. *Crit. Rev. Ther. Drug Carrier Syst.* 1998, 15:381-420.
[105] Vega E, Gamisans F, Garcia ML, Chauvet A, Lacoulonche F, Egea MA: PLGA Nanospheres for the Ocular Delivery of Flurbiprofen: Drug Release and Interactions. *Journal of Pharmaceutical Sciences.* 2008, 97:5306-5317.
[106] Agnihotri SM, Vavia PR: Diclofenac-loaded biopolymeric nanosuspensions for ophthalmic application. *Nanomedicine-Nanotechnology Biology and Medicine.* 2009, 5:90-95.
[107] Pignatello R, Bucolo C, Puglisi G: Ocular tolerability of Eudragit RS100 (R) and RL1009 (R) nanosuspensions as carriers for ophthalmic controlled drug delivery. *Journal of Pharmaceutical Sciences.* 2002, 91:2636-2641.
[108] Pignatello R, Bucolo C, Ferrara P, Maltese A, Puleo A, Puglisi G: Eudragit RS100 (R) nanosuspensions for the ophthalmic controlled delivery of ibuprofen. *European Journal of Pharmaceutical Sciences.* 2002, 16:53-61.
[109] Pignatello R, Bucolo C, Spedalieri G, Maltese A, Puglisi G: Flurbiprofen-loaded acrylate polymer nanosuspensions for ophthalmic application. *Biomaterials.* 2002, 23:3247-3255.
[110] Calvo P, SÃ˘nchez A, MartÃ-nez J, LÃłpez MI, Calonge M, Pastor JC, Alonso MJ: Polyester nanocapsules as new topical ocular delivery systems for cyclosporin A. *Pharmaceutical Research.* 1996, 13:311-315.
[111] Le Bourlais CA, Chevanne F, Turlin B, Acar L, Zia H, Sado PA, Needham TE, Leverge R: Effect of cyclosporine A formulations on

bovine corneal absorption: ex-vivo study. *J. Microencapsul.* 1997, 14: 457-467
[112] Yenice I, Mocan M, Palaska E, Bochot A, Bilensoy E, Vural I, Irkeç M, Hincal A: Hyaluronic acid coated poly-epsilon-caprolactone nanospheres deliver high concentrations of cyclosporine A into the cornea. *Exp. Eye Res.* 2008, 87:162-167.
[113] Lehr C-M, Bouwstra JA, Schacht EH, Junginger HE: In vitro evaluation of mucoadhesive properties of chitosan and some other natural polymers. *International Journal of Pharmaceutics.* 1992, 78:43-48.
[114] Zambito Y, Zaino C, Di Colo G: Effects of N-trimethylchitosan on transcellular and paracellular transcorneal drug transport. *European Journal of Pharmaceutics and Biopharmaceutics.* 2006, 64:16-25.
[115] Yuan XB, Li H, Yuan YB: Preparation of cholesterol-modified chitosan self-aggregated nanoparticles for delivery of drugs to ocular surface. *Carbohydrate Polymers.* 2006, 65:337-345.
[116] Calvo P, Remunán-López C, Vila-Jato JL, Alonso MJ: Novel hydrophilic chitosan-polyethylene oxide nanoparticles as protein carriers. *Journal of Applied Polymer Science.* 1997, 63:125-132.
[117] de Salamanca A, Diebold Y, Calonge M, Garcia-Vazquez C, Callejo S, Vila A, Alonso MJ: Chitosan nanoparticles as a potential drug delivery system for the ocular surface: toxicity, uptake mechanism and in vivo tolerance. *Invest. Ophthalmol. Vis. Sci.* 2006, 47:1416-1425.
[118] De Campos AM, Sanchez A, Alonso MJ: Chitosan nanoparticles: a new vehicle for the improvement of the delivery of drugs to the ocular surface. Application to cyclosporin A. *Int. J. Pharm.* 2001, 224:159-168.
[119] De Campos AM, Sanchez A, Gref R, Calvo P, Alonso MJ: The effect of a PEG versus a chitosan coating on the interaction of drug colloidal carriers with the ocular mucosa. *Eur. J. Pharm. Sci.* 2003, 20:73-81.
[120] Yuan XB, Yuan YB, Jiang W, Liu J, Tian EJ, Shun HM, Huang DH, Yuan XY, Li H, Sheng J: Preparation of rapamycin-loaded chitosan/PLA nanoparticles for immunosuppression in corneal transplantation. *International Journal of Pharmaceutics.* 2008, 349:241-248.
[121] Sandri G, Bonferoni MC, Gökçe EH, Ferrari F, Rossi S, Caramella C: Chitosan Associated Solid Lipid Nanoparticles: Assessement of Penetration Enhancement Properties Using RCE cell line. In *37th Controlled Release Society Annual Meeting & Exposition*; *18-23 July 2009; Copenhagen, Denmark.* 2009

[122] Diebold Y, Jarrin M, Saez V, Carvalho EL, Orea M, Calonge M, Seijo B, Alonso MJ: Ocular drug delivery by liposome-chitosan nanoparticle complexes (LCS-NP). *Biomaterials.* 2007, 28:1553-1564.

[123] Mehanna MM, Elmaradny HA, Samaha MW: Mucoadhesive liposomes as ocular delivery system: physical, microbiological, and in vivo assessment. *Drug Dev. Ind. Pharm.* 2009.

[124] Li N, Zhuang C, Wang M, Sun X, Nie S, Pan W: Liposome coated with low molecular weight chitosan and its potential use in ocular drug delivery. *Int. J. Pharm.* 2009.

[125] Souto EB, Müller RH: Lipid nanoparticles (SLN and NLC) for drug delivery. In *Nanoparticles for Pharmaceutical Applications.* Volume 01-2007. Edited by Domb AJ, Tabata Y, Ravi Kumar MNV, Farber S. Los Angeles, California: American Scientific Publishers; 2007: 103-122

[126] Cavalli R, Gasco MR, Chetoni P, Burgalassi S, Saettone MF: Solid lipid nanoparticles (SLN) as ocular delivery system for tobramycin. *Int. J. Pharm.* 2002, 238:241-245.

[127] Li X, Nie SF, Kong J, Li N, Ju CY, Pan WS: A controlled-release ocular delivery system for ibuprofen based on nanostructured lipid carriers. *International Journal of Pharmaceutics.* 2008, 363:177-182.

[128] Attama AA, Reichl S, Muller-Goymann CC: Diclofenac sodium delivery to the eye: In vitro evaluation of novel solid lipid nanoparticle formulation using human cornea construct. *International Journal of Pharmaceutics.* 2008, 355:307-313.

[129] Attama AA, Muller-Goymann CC: Investigation of surface-modified solid lipid nanocontainers formulated with a heterolipid-templated homolipid. *Int. J. Pharm.* 2007, 334:179-189.

[130] Cengiz E, Demirel M, Yazan Y: Ocular Fate of Cyclosporine-A with Solid Lipid Nanoparticles. In *6th World Meeting on Pharmaceutics, Biopharmaceutics and Pharmaceutical Technology*; *7-10 April 2008; Barcelona, Spain.* 2008

[131] Gökçe EH, Sandri G, Bonferoni MC, Rossi S, Ferrari F, Güneri T, Caramella C: Cyclosporine A loaded SLNs: Evaluation of cellular uptake and corneal cytotoxicity. *International Journal of Pharmaceutics.* 2008, 364:76-86.

[132] Niu M, Shi K, Sun Y, Wang J, Cui F: Preparation of CyA-loaded solid lipid nanoparticles and application on ocular preparations. *Journal of Drug Delivery Science and Technology.* 2008, 18:293-297.

[133] Başaran E, Demirel M, Sırmagül B, Yazan Y: Cyclosporine-A incorporated cationic solid lipid nanoparticles for ocular delivery. *J. Microencapsul.* 2009, doi:10.1080/02652040902846883.

[134] Niu M-m, Yu Y-w, Shi K, Zhang L-q, Lin W-h, Cui F-d: A novel solid lipid nanoparticles loaded in situ gel for CyA delivery and its lacrimal pharmacokinetics in rabbit tears *Journal of Shengyang Pharmaceutical university.* 2009, 26:507-511

[135] Shen J, Wang Y, Ping Q, Xiao Y, Huang X: Mucoadhesive effect of thiolated PEG stearate and its modified NLC for ocular drug delivery. *Journal of Controlled Release.* 2009, 137:217-223.

[136] Gökçe EH, Sandri G, Bonferoni MC, Güneri T, Caramella C: Freeze-drying of Cyclosporine A Loaded Solid Lipid Nanoparticles In *37th Controlled Release Society Annual Meeting & Exposition*; *18-23th July 2009; Copenhagen, Denmark.* 2009

[137] Samad A, Sultana Y, Aqil M: Liposomal Drug Delivery Systems: An Update Review. *Curr Drug Deliv* 2007, 4:297-305.

[138] Ebrahim S, Peyman GA, Lee PJ: Applications of liposomes in ophthalmology. *Survey of Ophthalmology.* 2005, 50:167-182.

[139] Sun KX, Wang AP, Huang LJ, Liang RC, Liu K: Preparation of diclofenac sodium liposomes and its ocular pharmacokinetics. *Yao Xue Xue Bao.* 2006, 41:1094-1098.

[140] Pleyer U, Lutz S, Jusko W, Nguyen K, Narawane M, Ruckert D, Mondino B, Lee V, K N: Ocular absorption of topically applied FK506 from liposomal and oil formulations in the rabbit eye [published erratum appears in Invest Ophthalmol Vis Sci 1993 Nov;34(12):3481]. *Invest. Ophthalmol. Vis. Sci.* 1993, 34:2737-2742.

[141] Dausch D, Lee S, Dausch S, Kim JC, Schwert G, Michelson W: Vergleichende Studie zur Therapie des Trockenen Auges bedingt durch Lipidphasenstörungen mit lipidhaltigen Tränenpräparaten [Comparative Study of Treatment of the Dry Eye Syndrome due to Disturbances of the Tear Film Lipid Layer with Lipid-Containing Tear Substitutes]. *Klin. Monatsbl. Augenheilkd.* 2006, 223:974-983.

[142] Khaireddin R, Schmidt KG: Vergleichende Untersuchung zur Therapie des evaporativen trockenen Auges [Comparative Investigation of Treatments for Evaporative Dry Eye]. *Klin. Monatsbl. Augenheilkd.* 2009.

[143] Craig JP, Purslow C, Murphy PJ, Wolffsohn JS: Effect Of A Liposomal Spray On The Preocular Tear Film. In *5th International Conference on*

the Tear Film & Ocular Surface: Basic Science and Clinical Relevance; Taormina, Sicily, Italy. 2007

[144] Oh C, Saville BA, Cheng Y-L, Rootman DS: A Compartmental Model for the Ocular Pharmacokinetics of Cyclosporine in Rabbits. *Pharm. Res.* 1995, 12:433-437.

[145] Yenice I, Mocan MC, Palaska E, Bochot A, Bilensoy E, Vural I, Irkec M, Hincal AA: Hyaluronic acid coated poly-epsilon-caprolactone nanospheres deliver high concentrations of cyclosporine A into the cornea. *Experimental Eye Research.* 2008, 87:162-167.

[146] Varia J, Dodiya S, Sawant K: Cyclosporine a loaded solid lipid nanoparticles: optimization of formulation, process variable and characterization. *Curr. Drug Deliv.* 2008, 5:64-69.

[147] Castelli F, Messina C, Pignatello R, Puglisi G: Effect of pH on diclofenac release from Eudragit RS100 (R) microparticles. A kinetic study by DSC. *Drug Delivery.* 2001, 8:173-177.

[148] Attama AA, Schicke BC, Paepenmuller T, Muller-Goymann CC: Solid lipid nanodispersions containing mixed lipid core and a polar heterolipid: Characterization. *European Journal of Pharmaceutics and Biopharmaceutics.* 2007, 67:48-57.

[149] Bucolo C, Maltese A, Puglisi G, Pignatello R: Enhanced ocular anti-inflammatory activity of Ibuprofen carried by an Eudragit RS100((R)) nanoparticle suspension. *Ophthalmic Research.* 2002, 34:319-323.

[150] Castelli F, Messina C, Sarpietro MG, Pignatello R, Puglisi G: Eudragit as controlled release system for anti-inflammatory drugs - A comparison between DSC and dialysis experiments. *Thermochimica Acta.* 2003, 400:227-234.

[151] Vega E, Egea MA, Valls O, Espina M, Garcia ML: Flurbiprofen loaded biodegradable nanoparticles for ophtalmic administration. *Journal of Pharmaceutical Sciences.* 2006, 95:2393-2405.

[152] Yamaguchi M, Ueda K, Isowaki A, Ohtori A, Takeuchi H, Ohguro N, Tojo K: Mucoadhesive Properties of Chitosan-Coated Ophthalmic Lipid Emulsion Containing Indomethacin in Tear Fluid. *Biological & Pharmaceutical Bulletin.* 2009, 32:1266-1271.

[153] Calvo P, Alonso MJ, Vila-Jato JL, Robinson JR: Improved Ocular Bioavailability of Indomethacin by Novel Ocular Drug Carriers. *Journal of Pharmacy and Pharmacology.* 1996, 48:1147-1152.

[154] Adibkia K, Shadbad MRS, Nokhodchi A, Javadzedeh A, Barzegar-Jalali M, Barar J, Mohammadi G, Omidi Y: Piroxicam nanoparticles for ocular delivery: Physicochemical characterization and implementation in

endotoxin-induced uveitis. *Journal of Drug Targeting.* 2007, 15:407-416.

Index

A

acetylcholine, 33
acid, 11, 18, 24, 25, 32, 33, 35, 36, 38, 44, 45, 49, 51, 53, 56, 59
acne, 53
acrylate, 55
acrylic acid, 49
acupuncture, 34, 54
additives, 26
adhesion, 19, 24
adhesive properties, 43
afferent nerve, 17
age, 18
aggression, 20
AIDS, 19
alcohol, 11
alcoholism, 19
alcohols, 25
allergic reaction, 26
ambroxol, 29
androgen, 18, 32
androgens, 20
anticholinergic, 23
anticholinergic effect, 23
anti-inflammatory drugs, 31, 53, 59
apoptosis, 20, 29
aqueous humor, 35
aqueous solutions, 24
aqueous suspension, 14

argon, 28
assessment, 37, 57
astringent, 24
atopic dermatitis, 19
atrophy, 19, 27
authors, 15
autoimmune disease, 30
availability, 35

B

bacteria, 18, 20, 24
bacterial conjunctivitis, 31
bacterial infection, 28
barriers, 34
beneficial effect, 33
binding, 20
binding globulin, 20
bioavailability, 14, 34, 35, 36, 37, 39, 40, 41, 43, 45
biocompatibility, 37
birth, 20
birth control, 20
blepharitis, 30, 53
blepharospasm, 33
blindness, 32
blood, 17, 38
boric acid, 25
brain, 17
breakdown, 19

buffer, 44
burning, 29

C

carrier, 15, 26, 36, 38, 43
castor oil, 36, 44
cataract, 31, 35
cell, 19, 20, 25, 30, 37, 40, 48, 56
cell culture, 40
cell death, 19, 20
cell line, 37, 56
cell lines, 37
cell surface, 19
cellular regulation, 18
cellulose, 24, 26
children, 53
cholesterol, 37, 56
chronic diseases, 31
chronic irritation, 29
circulation, 17, 38
clinical trials, 34, 50
coatings, 37, 45
cobalt, 21
collagen, 27, 51
complement, 30
compliance, 14, 23, 26
complications, 19, 27, 31, 32
components, 25, 32, 34
composition, 13, 19, 20, 24, 27, 38, 41
compounds, 25
concentration, 35, 36, 37, 38, 44, 45
condensation, 28
conjunctiva, 17, 18, 27, 28, 29, 31, 32, 36, 37, 44, 45
conjunctivitis, 31
connective tissue, 19
consensus, 49
contamination, 25, 33, 50
contraceptives, 18
control, 21, 33, 53
copolymers, 35, 49
cornea, 13, 14, 17, 18, 21, 24, 31, 32, 35, 36, 37, 38, 39, 44, 45, 56, 57, 59
corneal transplant, 56

corneal ulcer, 28, 30
correlation, 29
corticosteroids, 30, 52
costs, 41
covering, 28
crocodile, 54
cyclosporine, 14, 30, 36, 37, 38, 39, 40, 45, 52, 55, 56, 59
cytokines, 19, 20, 29, 48
cytomegalovirus, 19
cytotoxicity, 57

D

defects, 28, 31, 32
defence, 17, 24
deficiency, 18, 20, 48
deficit, 30
definition, 13
degradation, 37
dehydration, 19
delivery, 13, 14, 15, 34, 35, 36, 38, 39, 40, 49, 50, 55, 56, 57, 58, 59
Denmark, 56, 58
density, 30
deprivation, 20
desiccation, 17, 28
destruction, 18, 19
diabetes, 19
dialysis, 59
diapedesis, 19
differentiation, 18, 29, 32
diffusion, 24
discomfort, vii, 13, 25, 27, 28, 31, 49
disorder, 13, 19
dispersion, 14
division, 20
DNA, 54
dosage, vii, 13, 14, 26, 36
dose-response relationship, 30
drainage, 14, 23, 27, 28, 33, 54
drug carriers, 55
drug delivery, vii, 15, 26, 35, 37, 38, 39, 40, 43, 47, 49, 50, 55, 56, 57, 58
drug release, 35, 36, 41

drugs, 14, 29, 31, 34, 35, 36, 40, 43, 44, 56
dry eyes, 28, 33, 47, 48, 49
drying, 23, 32, 40, 58
DSC, 59
duration, 50

E

ears, 29
electrodes, 28
electrolyte, 26, 50
emulsions, 14, 30, 39
encapsulation, 15, 41
encouragement, 23
enlargement, 20
environment, 18, 20
environmental factors, 23
enzymes, 24
eosinophils, 19
epithelia, 20
epithelial cells, 17, 18, 19, 20, 21, 29, 32, 40, 48, 50
epithelium, 17, 19, 20, 28, 32, 39, 45, 48, 54
Epstein-Barr virus, 54
estrogen, 32, 53
etiology, 20
evaporation, 21, 28
evolution, 34
exposure, 13, 18

F

failure, 19
family, 19
fat, 39
fatigue, 21
FDA, 30
fibers, 21
flight, 13
fluid, 23, 24, 26, 27, 28
follicles, 17

G

ganglion, 17
gel, 41, 58
gelation, 37
gene, 19, 48
gene expression, 48
generation, 17
gland, 18, 20, 27, 29, 32, 48, 49, 50, 54
glasses, 23
glycol, 11, 38
goals, 23
goblet cells, 18, 20, 32, 49
groups, 37, 38, 39
growth, 30, 32, 39
growth factor, 30, 32

H

health, 18, 50
heat, 21, 28
height, 21
HIV, 54
HIV infection, 54
HLA, 33, 54
homeostasis, 20
hormone, 20
human leukocyte antigen, 33
humidity, 18, 23, 24, 28
hydrogels, vii, 14, 49
hydroxypropyl cellulose, 26, 50
hygiene, 31
hyperemia, 29
hypertension, 31
hypothyroidism, 19

I

iatrogenic, 25
ibuprofen, 35, 55, 57
ICAM, 19
ideal, 14, 24, 49
IFN, 19, 29
IL-6, 29

image, 38
immune response, 19
immunomodulation, 30
immunomodulatory, 30
immunosuppression, 56
implementation, 59
in vitro, 50
in vivo, 37, 40, 56, 57
indication, 32
infection, 31
infectious mononucleosis, 19
inflammation, vii, 18, 19, 20, 30, 34, 36, 41
inflammatory cells, 30
inflammatory disease, 31
injections, 33
injuries, 21, 23
injury, iv, 19
insertion, 27
instability, vii
integrity, 31
interaction, 37, 51, 56
intercellular adhesion molecule, 19
interval, 21
intraocular, 38
involution, 19
iris, 38
isolation, 19
Italy, 59

K

keratoconjunctivitis, vii, 13, 19, 30, 32, 47, 48, 50, 52, 53, 54

L

Langerhans cells, 17
lasers, 28
lens, 30, 32
lifetime, 13
limitation, 14
line, 24
lipids, 17, 20, 21, 24, 39
liposomes, 38, 40, 41, 57, 58

lubricants, 24, 27, 32
lymphocytes, 17, 20
lysozyme, 24, 34, 37

M

macrophages, 17
maintenance, 26
malnutrition, 18
management, vii, 13, 14, 23, 43
manipulation, 14
market, 25, 39, 41, 43
mast cells, 19
measures, 23, 24
medication, 29
Mediterranean, 29
melting, 20, 31, 53
menopause, 19
metabolism, 17
miosis, 35
model, 35
models, 39
moisture, 23
molecular weight, 37, 57
molecules, 19, 34
morbidity, 19
mucin, 18, 21, 34, 37, 45, 49
mucosa, 20, 35, 56
mucous membrane, 18
mucous membranes, 18
mucus, 25
multiple factors, 18

N

nanoparticles, 34, 35, 36, 37, 38, 39, 40, 43, 45, 49, 55, 56, 57, 58, 59
natural polymers, 56
nerve, 14, 17, 18, 30
nerve growth factor, 30
neural function, 19
nodules, 30
NSAIDs, 11, 31, 35, 39, 41, 43

O

objectives, 23
observations, 34
occlusion, 23, 27, 28, 33, 50, 51
octopus, 29
ocular diseases, 40
oil, 18, 36, 39, 58
olive oil, 36, 44
ophthalmologist, 19
optimization, 59
organic solvents, 37
ovariectomy, 19
ovaries, 20
oxide nanoparticles, 56
oxygen, 18

P

pain, 23, 31, 33
palliative, 23
paralysis, 33
parameters, 41
parotid, 27
particles, 15, 18, 37, 38, 39, 43
pathogenesis, 13, 20
pathology, 18, 51
pathophysiology, 47
pathways, 19
peptides, 41
perforation, 21, 53
permeation, 35, 38, 39, 40, 44, 45
pharmacokinetics, 58
pheochromocytoma, 19
phosphates, 26
phospholipids, 38, 41
photophobia, 21, 31
physiology, 47
placebo, 30, 52
plasma, 38
pollution, 18
polymer, 25, 34, 37, 55
polymer structure, 34
polymers, vii, 24, 25, 26, 35, 38, 55
polyvinyl alcohol, 24, 35, 45
Portugal, ix
potassium, 25
pregnancy, 19, 20
preservative, 25, 26, 36, 50
pressure, 37
production, 14, 18, 24, 27, 30, 33, 34, 39, 40, 50, 51, 53
production costs, 14
pro-inflammatory, 20, 29
proliferation, 32
proteins, 19, 21, 24
pruritus, 27
Pseudomonas aeruginosa, 25
PVA, 11, 44, 45

Q

quality of life, 13
quaternary ammonium, 25

R

range, 15
reason, 20
receptors, 19, 32, 53
recovery, 26
reflection, 21
refractive index, 14
regulation, 20
regulations, 33
relief, vii, 25, 28, 41, 54, 55
repair, 18
residues, 37
resistance, 33
retention, 24, 39, 44
retinol, 32, 47
risk, 33
rods, 26
room temperature, 39
rosacea, 31, 53

S

safety, 43, 49, 51, 52
saliva, 27
salivary glands, 29
salt, 35, 39
scores, 33
secretion, 17, 18, 20, 27, 28, 29, 31, 51
selecting, 38
sensation, 13, 14, 21, 25, 26, 27, 29, 50
serum, 32, 48, 53
severity, 24
sex, 20
sialic acid, 37
side effects, 14, 31, 38
signalling, 19
signs, 13, 21, 30, 31, 32, 33, 34
silicon, 27
skin, 19
smoke, 23
sodium, 26, 35, 36, 39, 52, 57, 58
sodium hydroxide, 26
solubility, 37
space, 14
speed, 13
stability, 24, 25, 33, 34, 37, 39, 41
stabilizers, 25
staphylococci, 53
stenosis, 27
steroids, 31, 48
Stevens-Johnson syndrome, 32, 53
storage, 41
strategies, 25
stratification, 20
stress, 47
stroma, 19
substitutes, 26
substitution, 24
Sun, 49, 57, 58
surface tension, 24
surfactant, 36
susceptibility, 33
swelling, 37
symptom, 33
symptoms, vii, 13, 18, 20, 21, 25, 30, 31, 32, 33, 34
synapse, 17
syndrome, vii, 13, 14, 18, 19, 20, 29, 31, 33, 34, 35, 36, 48, 49, 50, 54, 55
synthetic polymers, 34

T

T cell, 18, 47
T lymphocytes, 19
tamoxifen, 18
targets, 32
temperature, 20, 27, 37
terminals, 18
therapeutic approaches, vii
therapy, 23, 24, 27, 29, 30, 32, 34, 35, 40, 41, 51, 53
tissue, 13, 15, 19, 20, 29, 40, 44
TNF, 29
TNF-α, 29
toxicity, 27, 56
toxin, 18, 33, 54
traffic, 18
tranquilizers, 18
transparency, 14, 17
transplantation, 27
transport, 45, 56
trial, 30, 32, 51, 52
trigeminal nerve, 17, 20
triglycerides, 36
turnover, 27
typhoid, 18
typhoid fever, 18

U

ultrastructure, 26
uniform, 23
uveitis, 60

V

vasodilation, 29

viruses, 18, 34
viscosity, 25, 26, 35, 37
vision, vii, 14, 15, 21, 23, 25, 26
visual acuity, 24
vitamin A, 30, 32
vitamins, 33
vocational performance, 13

wind, 18, 21, 23
wound healing, 17, 38

xerophthalmia, 32, 33
xerostomia, 34, 54

water evaporation, 51
wetting, 24